Help! I'm a Caregiver

A Book of Helps, Comfort, Insights, and Encouragement

Ernest M. Tegeder

ISBN 978-1-0980-8633-6 (paperback)
ISBN 978-1-0980-8634-3 (digital)

Christian Faith Publishing, Inc.
832 Park Avenue
Meadville, PA 16335
www.christianfaithpublishing.com

Printed in the United States of America

I dedicate this book to my Lord and Savior Jesus Christ,
and my dear wife, Barbara, the love of my life,
for whom it is now my privilege to be her caregiver.

Contents

Preface

This book has been written as a help, guide, encouragement, and hurrah for anyone who finds they have been assigned to care for a child, mate, elderly parent, or perhaps in a professional capacity.

You will discover very quickly that caregiving is no easy task, and it involves many facets. It will tax everything about you from your strength to your emotions, patience, spiritual strength, and right down to your very character.

This book will also not pull punches and will confront head-on all the issues you will face and encounter. In all likelihood, some of the issues you will or must confront you may find troublesome or embarrassing, in that certain thoughts and feelings may arise that you wish didn't. Confronting them will help you deal with your state of mind.

Lastly, this book is written from a godly Christian perspective—which, if you are one, you will welcome. And if you are not, you may be led and drawn by it to a relationship with Jesus Christ, our loving God and Creator.

Introduction

It's been said we come into this world needing lots of care and we generally leave it the same way. Therefore caregiving is a necessity, but it is something more. It is an expression of reality combined with love. The reality is that the human condition we pass through puts all of us in need of care at some point and the love part is how and who gives it and how it is given.

The chapters, and how they are presented, introduce one to the various aspects of caregiving plus, in some cases, present information particularly aimed at a specific disease. I encourage you to read all the chapters, not just the ones you might cherry-pick as applying to your particular situation, as there are crossover points that connect many, if not all of them. This is especially true if you intend to be a professional caregiver.

And you might find it painful to confront some of the points brought up, and they may prove emotionally hard and tearful. This is understood, and one should not be ashamed of shedding a few as life—this veil of tears—does have its sad moments and seasons.

But caregiving is one of those things that will cause you to see life differently as you begin to understand we are all connected, and we are called to serve one another in love and compassion. Further, God states that what you do for someone else is actually done for God Himself! This principle is one of the prime directives of life and embodies the meaning of the parable of the Good Samaritan.

We really are called to be a help and a blessing, and when we operate this way, we are fulfilling the second great commandment to love one's neighbor as one's self.

And as it turns out in reality, everyone is our neighbor in God's sight.

Caregiving as a Profession

Caregiving as a profession exists because it is needed, and it cannot always be provided by a family member. The reasons are obvious as there may be no family member available or the nature of the caregiving may require training and physical strength beyond the available member's capabilities. Or the member available might have to hold a job outside the home.

Professional caregiving runs the gamut from deep bedside care of a hospice or near-hospice level to physical therapy needed to help one keep operating on a physical level in day-to-day living.

It can be needed due to illness recovery or ongoing debilitation or recovery from injury or accident. Looking at this from a Christian perspective, our present bodies are subject to injury, illness, and deterioration due to aging.

This is the physical side of things, but there is also the emotional and mental as well. Someone who can no longer perform what they once could will likely be impacted in some way mentally or emotionally or both. As a caregiver, this must be recognized and managed as part of ongoing care.

An example of this would be an athlete whose skill has declined to a point they can no longer perform on a competitive level even though they might not be what one would call disabled. But because of whatever injury or illness or age their competitive decline no longer affords them the "notice" or sports coverage once enjoyed and this often leads to emotional problems. What once brought that individual fame and high income no longer does, and this then can impact the individual's identity and self-worth. It's not that the athlete is in need of therapy for a career-ending injury as much as counseling and acceptance of this new phase in their life.

This is a mild example, of course, and most of us do not reach a level of that kind of fame and notice, but as time goes on, we all face decline and adjustments in some aspects of our abilities at the least. And the caregiver themselves may someday require the very care they are now giving. Even doctors who care and cure must acknowledge their own mortality. Or to put it another way, even doctors get sick.

So as a caregiver, you might find the larger of the two aspects of care required, *physical* or *emotional/spiritual* to be the latter and may be even more impactful than the physical side. What your own personage brings to the relationship may be even more impactful in the care and healing process than even the physical side of it.

To ignore the emotional/spiritual nature of a human being is not to recognize the fact that we are body, mind, and spirit, and as such, each one impacts the other.

What then are the things that a caregiver can bring to the patient? They are cheerfulness, humor, hopefulness, respect, concern and interest, as well as developing creative ways to express these things. All of them, in reality, have a spiritual dimension side attached. Getting to know the patient and what makes them up as a person conveys to them that they are still viable as a person and have something to share and give. This is very healing, and many a caregiver will attest to receiving as much from a patient as they have given in care.

However, as warm and fuzzy and good feeling as this is, there is a downside to it that one must be aware of. Caregiving is one of those professions that can be a downer for the giver. It is not always easy to walk away from the job each day and not bring some of it home. Or if it is the home where you live, keeping it home and internalizing it. Like policework, military, and a few other professions, your job can impact your life at home or away from the job. In the later chapters, we will deal with how to maintain your own healthy outlook. But before we leave this matter for the moment, recognize it is not wrong to have troubling thoughts or emotions—and that having them does not make you a bad person. In fact, it is more likely you will experience troubling thoughts, and we'll deal with that later on.

When I was in my final semester of undergrad college, having already secured a teaching position (and a waiting job in September), a course was required called Teacher in School and Community that dealt with all aspects of exactly what the course title indicated. Some of them came as a surprise, one of which was preparing for retirement. Really? And I hadn't even taught my first day! Well, I realized there was more to the job than met the eye. And now having been retired with thirty-seven years of public school music education behind me, I could add a few things of my own.

Did the course discourage me in any way? Not really. I was idealistic and anxious to teach. However, all jobs have negatives and positives, and it's good to be aware of them ahead of time. And from my vantage point now, would I, if just starting out, elect to go into public education? Well, it's a different ballgame now (and world) and I think much tougher—mainly from the societal and social aspects—and I'm glad I don't have to make that decision. For me, the years I taught were rewarding, all things considered. But one thing is certain, teachers, like caregivers, will always be needed.

Doctors—The Caregiver's Partner

Doctors—where would we be without them? It's been said medicine is an art as well as a science. I believe this to be true as there are so many differences patient to patient and people in general. We all don't develop the same illnesses. But before any treatment can begin, there must first be a diagnosis. A broken arm or leg, cut, abrasion is obvious, but when it comes to internal medicine, it is a different story.

The body has many systems that must all interact digestion, endocrine, pulmonary, vascular to list the main ones. Within these systems are subsystems that must interact properly. When a physician orders blood tests, he/she is looking at the indicators and parameters to see if the various systems chemical and otherwise fall between accepted norms. Based on these and patient blood history, the physician will make decisions and diagnosis as to the patients' condition treatment, medications, further tests, and may recommend a specialist.

Once treatment decisions have been made and medications prescribed the "torch," so to speak, passes to the caregiver who then must supervise and see that the meds are gotten and administered properly, and if physical therapy is recommended, seeing to it that the patient follows through with that assigned to homework.

One easily sees that caregiving begins with the physician and proper caregiving cannot take place until the patient is properly diagnosed, and a caregiver cannot prescribe medication or treatment.

Sometimes the human body is likened to a machine of sorts, and seeing a physician might be likened to take one's car, which is not running properly to a mechanic. If you have a good mechanic, be thankful and if you have a good doctor, a thousand times more so.

Yes, if you've ever been helped or cured through a doctor's care you should be thankful—we all should. Practicing medicine today is not easy, nor is it easy becoming a physician. Most people know this, that it takes years to become one—and that is to get to the point of residency. When one successfully completes that, one can be considered a physician. But a good doctor will tell you the learning is just getting started and never really stops.

The public, though, usually has two basic questions regarding medicine today, The first being why are there so many specialties? And the second, why are there so many tests?

The answer to the first is that as medicine has advanced; it becomes quite difficult to know everything about everything. All specialties have nuances of diagnosis and treatment, not to mention keeping up on the latest in one's field. And speaking of a nuance. It was a foot doctor who spotted a symptom of Parkinson's in my wife's stiffening and cramping toes. This was not the doctor's field, but his observation and leading proved to be correct.

And in answer to the second point, better for the patient to have one too many tests rather than a missed diagnosis. Plus, while this might sound a bit humorous, there is always a lawyer ready to jump on the case. This does the physician's reputation no good.

On this point, doctors must carry a very high malpractice insurance premium in the event of a misdiagnosis and/or treatment. Doctors are human too, and it can happen. But it is always to the patient's benefit to have any test the doctor feels is necessary. And running a practice is not easy as you have the expenses of staff, equipment, and that insurance we just mentioned

All this is something most patients, perhaps, are not aware of or not give it much thought. But a practice is not just patients; it is an "office of medicine" that must be run like a business and, as such, comes with its supply of headaches. Some doctors have left practice because of it. Those that remain should be applauded.

And before we close this chapter, we want and need to cite all doctors and specialists. And that includes dentists; dental surgeons; eye, ear, nose, and throat specialist; specialists of the skeletal regions (back, spine, knees, hands, and feet, and the vascular system), as well as all surgeons and anesthesiologists performing procedures in these areas as well as those internal. As you can see, that takes in a lot of territory, but we must also include the assistants, the hospitals, and surgical centers and last but not least, pharmacists and paramedical.

There is much involved in healthcare, and so often, we never think about what's involved in maintaining it. Even the walk-in centers deserve mention as sometimes it is the only place immediate care can be received. And of course, that includes the ER.

So a final hats off to all who take care of us, medically speaking, and to the researchers who are responsible for the advances in medicine.

Physical Therapists—
Caregivers Also

Physical therapists, in my opinion, are the unsung heroes of caregiving. They are the ones who come to grips with and confront the physical disabilities patients come to them with. Their job is to assess the level of disability and/or pain and start to map out what moves separately or in combination will rehabilitate the patient. In this sense, they are the first-line defense, physically speaking.

They are also diplomats in a sense because they often encounter resistance from a patient who complains of pain when asked to perform a movement. So the therapist has to encourage the patient to try but at the same time know and sense how far the patient can be pushed—not far enough, no progress, too far, patient discouragement and fear of pain or failure. The therapist then treads a fine line between push and stopping short of negative result.

The therapists I've observed are very good at this, and when my wife was finished with a session, she always walked and moved better than when she went in that day.

A good part of that was the personalities of the therapists and their expertise and sensitivity to where the patient was that day or overall.

Watching other patients arrive for their sessions, I've observed that if they were regulars, they seemed happy to be there and were looking forward to the session.

I've also noted new patients, and you can sense a bit of apprehension, but several sessions later, they seemed more relaxed and, again, happy to be going into another session.

I'm sure many a patient has realized they could do more than they thought—and that might be the biggest testimony to the work of the therapists. When the patient goes home thinking, "I can do more than I thought I could" or "This part of me that was stiff and hurting is now feeling a lot better" or still "I'm able to move about better now," well, for this, you can thank a therapist!

First Responders and ER Personnel—The Ultimate Caregivers

At first thought, first responders and ER personnel might not strike one as caregiving per se. But many owe their lives to these brave, dedicated men and women who deal with the worst of physical emergencies and trauma.

In my young days as senior in high school contemplating what career choice to make, one of my considerations was the New Jersey State Police. In fact, I was in the process of prequalifying for it through the NJ Boys State Program sponsored by the American Legion and administered through NJ high schools. Law enforcement greatly interested me as I saw it as a very patriotic American occupation. "To protect and serve" was my understanding and motivation. And being analytical by nature (plus a good shot), I felt I could handle the job, especially on the investigations side.

As it turned out, one of my high school teachers (teaching civics and history) was retired state police and was able to arrange for the then head of the state police—a Colonel Savage (and apt name for him as to his demeanor and appearance) to give the candidates and the student body a lecture. I assure you he pulled no punches. He was fiercely serious and proud of the force and its standards.

Once he finished explaining the rigid physical standards (it didn't sound like anyone could meet them), he went on to explain accident investigation. The scenes he described and the films a candidate would have to view were so horrible (and I'll decline to describe any) one had to wonder why anyone would take this job. He went on to say many candidates couldn't handle this and some would faint and throw up. One would have thought he was trying to discourage all candidates right off the bat.

But he made it clear the state police is very tough and for good reason. It gave ample meaning to the phrase "an awful job but someone has to do it."

I won't say this lecture discouraged me, but I did choose music over state police or astrophysics. However, I maintain great interest and respect for the state police having two other family members who joined the force, as well as respect and admiration for fire and emergency responders—and well, we all should. They live with danger and psychological pressure daily as do their families.

EMT responders are usually the first medical and comfort treatment and assurance a sick or injured individual receives and well as their families—plus good driving skills to get the patient to the ER as quickly and safely as possible.

Stages (Levels) of Caregiving

If you are considering caregiving as a profession or are new to it, either as a professional or family member who must now be one, it's good to be aware of what you will likely encounter. They will be listed in order of severity and duration.

1. Mild/temporary. Usually the result of injury or surgery where the convalescent period or debilitation that has resulted, the patient requires some assistance in daily living. Walking or driving may not be possible, but the healing process is relatively short. Often sports injuries come under this heading. Crutches or a wheelchair or walking cast may be involved.

2. Extended/prolonged. Much the same as mild/temporary but the recovery from the injury or surgery debilitation is longer due to the nature of, for example, injuries to back or both legs and generally necessitating a wheelchair. However, prognosis is good for returning to full abilities and function. Some assistance in dressing and undressing may be required.

3. Ongoing mild/permanent. Injury or illness is causing loss of abilities or function and daily living requires assistance, but the patient is ambulatory for the most part but may require help dressing, bathing, or cooking meals, or doing errands (banking, shopping, etc.) This level is often termed *assisted living*. While the patient with this level of care can often maintain a good life or living attitude and enjoyment, they will always need this level of care. Parkinson's patients often fall into this category.

4. Senior care. At this point, the patient requires assistance to do most everything, and while this can be much like the extended care category, it is usually required of a patient in declining health.
5. Hospice. In the final stages of life (days, weeks, sometimes months), most all things must be done for the patient, but the prime need is to keep the patient comfortable and comforted.

How one regards physical death depends on one's spiritual perspective. But one must understand "it is appointed to man once to die and then the judgement," so in that sense, we are assigned to that eventuality as a result of "the fall." It is a comfort, however, to know what God has done about this, and one must be assured death is not the end, rather a transition. But to those who remain, it is a separation.

Families in this modern age are often separated by great distances and circumstances and may not be able to be constantly available for and to the patient. Here, the caregiver is often put in the role of liaison to other family and officials. A special role to be sure but not an easy one and those specializing in hospice care understand this. But nonetheless, it is a special calling in caregiving and not everyone is equipped to handle this.

Devices and Apparatus Used in Caregiving

Because caregiving involves disability temporary or otherwise, there have been developed over time apparatus and implements to help the patient remain as ambulatory as possible and/or for the caregiver to assist in maintaining function and mobility.

We'll list them and then describe their use and functions: canes, crutches, wheelchairs (powered and nonpowered), braces, walkers, handrails and grabs, raised toilet seats, call devices, shower seats and low-entry tubs, and specialized vehicles (that can be self-driven or equipped with a lift to accept a wheelchair).

People with a disability may and usually will require some, if not all, of these, and as a caregiver, you may be responsible for assisting in their use and maintenance.

1. *Cane.* Simply a more developed and refined walking stick. Essentially, a cane allows the upper body to help support what the lower body or balance cannot do completely or reliably. It establishes a three-point balance base to assist in standing still, movement (walking), or getting up from a chair. The newest ones can be gotten with a three- or four-point (foot) base so that it can stand by itself and give a more solid feeling of support. And there is even a tall cane configured for assisting climb standing from a chair, having specially curved handle and grips. A cane can assist also in mild foot or leg surgery or injury healing and may be combined with a walking cast.

2.   *Crutches.* When the leg injury is too severe or extensive, and weight must be kept completely off, a cane may not be enough, and crutches will be necessary. It may take the user some time and instruction to get used to their use, and the caregiver must assist to guard against falls. And they can be somewhat of a nuisance to handle, store, and travel with. However, both cane and crutches can allow the patient to remain ambulatory. But note, crutches can be hard to use in confined living quarters and are not good for elderly patients who may lack the upper body strength to use them or use them safely. In general, though, the more athletic the patient naturally, the quicker they will tend to adapt to their use.

3.   *Wheelchairs.* When the patient cannot walk or should not walk during healing or has very poor balance or leg impairment of any kind, a wheelchair is the only recourse. Obviously more expensive than cane or crutches but very effective and necessary in these circumstances. If the patient is living at home, one's quarters must be equipped with a ramp to enter or exit if there are steps involved. In an apartment building, elevators can provide this. But many homes have steps, and for one person without help to enter or exit, a ramp is a must. In bad weather, the tires can track in mud and other debris—often a cleaning job for the caregiver. And though they can fold, they can be cumbersome to take in and out of a vehicle, another job for the caregiver as well as seeing to maintain lubrication on moving parts. For many patients though, it is the only way to remain ambulatory.

4.   *Walker.* One might classify this device as a lightweight wheelchair, but one that is used in an upright position allowing the patient to walk or move about. This is very helpful for patients who have poor strength and balance. Some are foldable and come in different styles and config-urations from basic to more elaborate with seats and back rests (a good idea to have) and can even be gotten with fold-

24

ing footrests so it can double as a lightweight wheelchair. The prices range from $50 for a basic one to $200 or more for a more elaborate one. However, it is recommended that the one purchased have four wheels (and not two sliders on the other two legs) and hand brakes, as this provides more safety and stability on ramps or inclines. Models with two sliders (sometimes capped with tennis balls) are not recommended for rough surfaces like cement, which can result in grabbing causing instability and falls. Also these models do not come with brakes, so they are extremely basic. Finally, walkers, like wheelchairs, can be difficult to negotiate in tight cramped areas and may require reconfiguring furniture plus lots of supervision until operations feels secure by the patient. And one last point, the three-wheel models offer more maneuverability in tight quarters but a sacrifice for the greater stability of the four-wheel models.

5. *Motorized wheelchairs.* These operate electrically and can and do cost upward of $2,000. If the patient has little to no strength or coordination to operate a standard wheelchair, then one with a motor can be the answer. However, the user must have hand control as switches and toggles control what it does and how it moves and at what speed. Instruction will be required before it will be safe to use by the patient and may not be suitable for the very elderly. And though you may see one on occasion going down the side of the street or road, this is not a recommended safe use. On a limited block, using the sidewalk is OK but not in the street!

6. *Motorized scooter chairs.* The next level of a motorized chair is the larger, heavier version, which can be used indoors (if room permits) or outdoors and is equipped with larger pneumatic tires. You may even have on occasion seen one going down the road close to the shoulder. Not recommended though for use in this way due to safety concerns. A user may insist they have control and feel safe. But they cannot maneuver quickly enough to get out of harm's way,

and sitting so low to the ground, they are not always able to be seen by motorists. These are best kept to sidewalks and senior living complexes. And these are expensive at more than $5,000, and being larger, they are not well suited for indoor use, unless one has a very large open floor layout.

7. *Specially equipped vehicles.* Usually vans, these vehicles are equipped with a lift that allows a person in a wheelchair to enter the vehicle and move to the driver's position while still in the chair (in this case, the patient must still be skilled and ambulatory to use a vehicle like this in this way; otherwise, it is to let the patient in and out for transport with a designated driver—usually the caregiver.) If driven by the patient while still in the wheelchair, the controls are configured to be hand operated as the feet cannot be employed. A patient able to use and operate such a vehicle is usually not in need of all but minimal caregiving, but it is mentioned to provide a complete picture of all that is available for the handicapped.

Very expensive at the price of $60,000 to $70,000 (unless one can find a used one), they can allow an individual to remain mobile and continue to earn a living. And if the patient is retired, these vehicles can keep patient from becoming house-bound. But these vehicles can be configured, as has been mentioned, with a lift to accept someone in a wheelchair who needs caregiving but is not driving. Sometimes this is the only way to get a patient to the doctor or for physical therapy. It does make transporting them so much easier. However, beyond the initial expense, the lift system must be maintained by someone qualified—an additional expense and time spent to bring it to the technician, if one does not make house calls.

8. *Handrails and grabs.* These come in several colors, finishes, and lengths. They are particularly useful at bedside and in the bathroom to assist the patient in getting up and standing until balance and stability has been achieved. But they also provide support and stability when the patient is try-

ing to sit. Also don't neglect to have them installed in the shower. These though will often require a skilled installer, particularly in the shower area when tile must be drilled.

9. *Raised toilet seats.* Along the lines of stability, sitting down or getting up from the toilet can have difficulties. A toilet five or so inches higher than average or usual makes the task easier and potentially less embarrassing for the patient. They come in various forms and configurations and are relatively inexpensive, and they merely fit down on top of the existing toilet seat with no tools required. A seat raiser should be on every floor the patient spends time. Finally, in addition to the seat riser, side lift handles should be part of the package and are available separately and are compatible with the seat riser. I have found both are really necessary.

10. *Shower seats and low-entry tubs.* A shower seat is a good investment for a patient with poor balance, and they are not expensive. They can be gotten or ordered (like most items) at your local surgical supply, if you have one. Low-entry tubs are a good idea if you can afford one and if you were going to remodel anyway. But be prepared for sticker shock as they are expensive for a number of reasons as remodeling involves demolition first, and because of the extreme weight of a walk-in tub filled, the framing structure in that area will have to be beefed up. You are talking about 1,000 to 2,000 lbs. when filled and with a person! Many times in an older home, the floor joists may be inadequate but can usually be reinforced. However, they can be most useful and therapeutic and can be gotten with or without jet massage. In the later versions, there is the added expense of a pump and wiring, therefore needing an electrician, which is usually provided by the installer.

11. *Call devices (pendants).* If the patient spends any time alone, this device can be a lifesaver. Falls, strokes, heart attacks, episodes, etc. can happen anytime, and the sooner help arrives, the better the patient's chances.

And finally, try to configure the patient's residence with as few obstacles as possible that can result in falls, as this is the number 1 patient hazard. Floor items such as rugs or stick-out table legs are the most common hazard. But tripping over a pet can be another and is sometimes overlooked. Pets are important, and the patient must be made aware to check where they step. It's noticed many times the patient will look around the room as they move but often do not look down and are sometimes easily distracted by what's around them, and this is most true when a patient has a hallucination, as in Parkinson's or Alzheimer's.

Also discourage the patient from standing on boxes and chairs to reach needed or wanted items. Better to let the caregiver get it.

Outfitting a home for a patient then can be a complex and expensive proposition and not all the items recommended may be affordable. Certain insurances cover some of the items, and this must be determined on an individual basis. But the more that can be done as needed can make the environment and daily life safer and easier for patient and caregiver.

The Finances of Caregiving

A household, which is now a caregiving environment, will find it is operating under a different set of financial circumstances. I am particularly directing this chapter to couples where one is the caregiver. This is mostly the case with senior couples as in their case, the disabilities, whatever they are, tend to be ongoing. Not to put a downer on that, but the illnesses and ailments seniors tend to get are, for the most part, ongoing.

A couple in this situation will find that their day-to-day life is different than before, both in activities and finances. One of the big items in this category is meals and food expenditures. Many household expenses do not change, like electric bills, insurances, heating costs, etc. But when it comes to meals, there tends to be a big change. My wife and I live in an area heavily populated with seniors, and we've noticed they eat out a lot (as do we). There are a number of reasons for this. Perhaps the caregiver is not a good cook nor wants to be. Cooking is messy, and you always have cleanup afterward. It's pleasant to eat out, and for some couples, it's perhaps the only change in environment and scenery they receive on a regular basis. It's a good place to enjoy friends, or the tasks in caregiving do not allow for creative cooking, shopping, and food storage.

Those are some of the main reasons. However, eating out can be expensive. There are ways to lessen the impact and still eat well.

First, look for coupons, like buy one dinner and the other is half price. Eat at places that give large portions and eat half and take the other half home for another meal (we do that a lot, and it works well). Second, make a list of the places to eat that offer the best value. Third, eat your main meal midday and keep breakfast and supper light. This is good for the waistline. Fourth, keep some food at home that is easy to prepare such as beans, canned soup, yogurt, and even hot dogs for a change of pace. Fifth, don't neglect fruits and don't neglect whole grains and other foods that help maintain regularity. Sixth, milk and eggs are great foods, and the most recent studies indicate we should all be eating more eggs to get, among other things, that vital Vitamin D for our immune systems. Seventh, try not to buy items you don't need. In our household, we go through a lot of paper towels and paper plates. These are handy but try to buy the cheapest. Eighth, try to use your leftovers but watch for spoilage. It's easy to lose track. If you bring some home from a restaurant, put a date on the box and the name of whose portion it was.

Generally, in our area, our monthly food budget is around $900 a month trying to stay at $30 per day. Special occasions sometimes upset that or just getting bored with the usual. But food is important and an expensive item, even for two people. So you'll have to watch that food budget and try to be as creative as possible.

The Emotional Aspects
of Caregiving

Emotions were created by God that we might feel deeply and have a deep awareness of what we are doing or involved in, a deeper life dimension, so to speak.

Plus emotions operate on many different levels. Is waxing a car an emotional experience? Or is gardening? How about cooking? Just to name a few. All these things have an emotion of satisfaction attached to them. There's something about a waxed beautiful paint job that satisfies and something about a scratch or a dent that horrifies.

Yes, and an adverse emotional reaction can ruin one's day, and if persistent enough, it can ruin a day, week, month, or one's life. Controlling one's emotions and learning to do so is important. And it is of utmost importance in caregiving. You aren't a whole lot of help to your charge if you are down and you transfer this through your emotions to them. Likewise, when you're with others and with family, downer emotions brought home from work are not good as well.

Well, we're not perfect as human beings, and we will slip up from time to time. The question is, how can we maintain a generally healthy emotional state in caregiving? Since we don't come equipped with an On and Off switch for various things, we have to learn to do this from within.

The first step is to constantly remind yourself of the what and the why you are doing caregiving. You are there to help someone and not become emotionally hurt yourself. You'll be a better caregiver if you are maintained in better emotional health.

The second step is dispassion or, more correctly, a dispassionate attitude. It's not that you don't care, but it is not you that needs the care you're giving. In short, don't take the job home. Do your job to the best of your ability and then go home. (The exception here is if you are the caregiver for a spouse, child, parent, or relative living with you. If this is the case, emotional release has to be dealt with differently, which we will do in a subsequent chapter.)

Third, outside of work, keep doing and in touch with the things that relax and satisfy. And that could be hobbies, friends, a sport, cooking, reading, music, art, cleaning, gardening—whatever provides that sense of satisfaction and well-being. In short, maintaining an interest and zest for life.

Fourth, but not last, keep in touch with God and don't neglect your spiritual life. Keep in mind that He loves and cares for the person in your charge but also for you just as much. You just happen, at the moment, to be on a different side of the physical in life's journey. We are not in a frozen moment in time but an ongoing journey of development. So whatever God gives you to do at any moment in time, try to do it well as unto Him. "So that I may boldly say the Lord is my helper" (Hebrews 13:6).

Another scripture from Philippians 2:4 that helps is this: "Look not only on your own things [life concerns] but on the things of others" (their concerns, interests, and dreams). While it is difficult to comprehend an all-powerful, all-present, omniscient God, you, in reality, have 100 percent of God's care and attention at all times—and so does the person you're caring for. How many are aware and take advantage of this truth?

As believers, we all need to understand that this state of existence is temporary, and there will be, in God's good time, a full restoration. And while this life tires and wears us out, there is an ultimate good (very good—in fact, glorious) outcome.

Staying focused on these things will make you a great caregiver and keep you solid and grounded as well.

So one can quickly and easily see things that can bring a patient down and how some appropriate humor may help the situation. Someone using a walker—especially new at it—might find a remark,

"Now this is a very fast walker so be sure to signal when merging into traffic!" Or "Someday when I might need one, I'm going to decorate it with streamers on the handles and a racoon tail!" One of my wife's therapists used a catchy phrase to help her remember the best posture position when rising from a chair which went like this: "Remember, nose over toes." The comments must fit the chemistry and the occasion, and comments "male to male," "male to female," "female to male," and "female to female" will, of course, vary and should fit the occasion and be in good taste. "I see you're complaining better today" would not be (although there may be days you would want to exclaim that).

Some individuals are naturally quick on their feet, so to speak, with the quip or the comment. If you are one of these, you are well equipped to interject and use humor. But if you are not naturally this way, don't worry or feel you have to force the issue or study joke books, as you can still employ the second weapon—cheerfulness combined with a caring attitude. This can be as effective as humor; sometimes even more so.

And then there's patient rapport. As you build this relationship, you will develop a better sense of what and when to inject something humorous. And you may find yourself caring for someone who, despite their disability, are nevertheless humorous themselves. A patient like this makes the job easier, of course, and they might turn out to be the one cheering you up! Not the first time this has happened. There are so many variables and possibilities, but as a professional, one needs to become aware and attuned to them.

Perhaps for a caregiver, the hardest of days to do one's job is when you don't feel quite up to it and maybe bringing a problem from home or one's own life. We all have those days. Many a day like this has started badly but ended well—and sometimes not. These are especially the times to ask for God's helping hand. Don't forget, He's the ultimate caregiver.

Humor and Cheerfulness

One of the most important qualities and aspects to maintain is a sense of humor and cheerfulness, and there are many reasons this is the case.

Humor is one of the greatest diffusers of emotional tension there is. A patient in need of caregiving, regardless of the need level, is not likely to be cheerful or in anything close to an upbeat state—particularly if there is pain involved (although there are exceptions). But sometimes, something humorous injected into the situation can help move the patient through the difficulty.

It is not that you have to be constantly cracking jokes or making cute remarks but rather learning to inject something of humor into the situation which can greatly help. However, trying too hard to be funny, and trying too frequently, will seem strained and contrived. So then balance and timing are called for. Or as we say in performance, timing is everything.

In this regard, getting to know one's patient's personality can help. You may encounter one that seems to have no reception or concept of the humor you're using or perhaps, as we say, has no sense of humor. If this is the case, one must be careful as the humor you're trying to inject may have the opposite effect. However, before you conclude that you're just perhaps dealing with a grouch, consider and assess the circumstances the patient is dealing with. In other words, put yourself in their shoes for a moment.

Some people suffer in silence, and some do not. Listen to the vocal reactions of the patient and what they're trying to express. Yes, you might be caring for a complainer but listen to what they're complaining about. Example, if you're caring for a young male or father, he may be feeling inadequate now as a provider, earner, and expressing the remorse or loss (even if temporary) of their strong male role. If it's a female mother who, at the moment, cannot do for her family and is frustrated by her disabled state and, in addition, may be feeling that she is unattractive to her husband and is fearing he may cease loving her. Add age to this at various points and stages of life, and you begin to grasp the mental and emotional side of what patients needing care are experiencing.

Elder Caregiving

Caring for an elderly person has different aspects to it than caring for one who is young or middle age.

To begin with, an elderly person may have greater incapacities and perhaps pain to go along with this. One of the biggest mental/ emotional aspects to consider and be aware of is the fact that the individual may no longer be able to do things they once could plus the loss of independence—no small item when you have lost it. Not being able to drive can be a big contributor to this. Most individuals do not like or enjoy being dependent, and this can or will affect their mood, demeanor, sleep, appetite, and in extreme cases, the will to live or just to go on.

Knowing this and confronting it presents many challenges for a caregiver—most particularly if the one being cared for is one's mate. But more on that in a later chapter.

An elderly person presents a different set of challenges and needs, from help in dressing and undressing to lavatory assistance and bathing assistance to help eating and managing their food (cutting, for example) to just moving about (perhaps with the aid of a walker or being wheelchair bound). General physical and vocal weakness may be present. But in general, the older and more debilitated the person, the more extreme and constant care will be needed.

We often rate things on a scale from 1 to 10. If we do it for caregiving, the scale might be something like this: 1–3 mild care, with little physical help needed; 4–7 more debilitation physically, emotionally, and mentally; 8–9 more extreme and constant care needed; and 10 the hospice state.

Even though the elderly present more intense caregiving needs, they have a lifetime of memories, experiences, and wisdom to share.

When growing up (age eleven to twelve), I was introduced to our neighbor's elderly mother whom they called Dranny. Even though bedridden, she was mentally razor-sharp and possessed much wisdom and knowledge. I spent many hours at her bedside visiting and absorbing her wisdom and loving every minute of it. And she was a big influence and contributor in the forming of my own character.

Not every elderly patient may be like this, but if you have the good fortune to be assigned to one, you are and will be greatly blessed.

Listening—Being a Good Listener

Another very important quality to have and employ is being a good listener. All patients will be communicating something in some way. These may run the gamut from just complaining or lamenting to expressing pain, regret, disappointment, frustration, anxiety, fear, dementia to just being very talkative and perhaps relating many life stories and experiences.

As you will likely be spending much time with the patient, being a good listener builds rapport and a good relationship, and that opens the door to being a help, encourager, comforter, and in some cases, receiving the same in return.

In general, women tend to be more talkative and have more need to communicate and express what they are feeling verbally. As mothers and nurturers, this is a godly built in quality. Also it tends to get things out in the open.

Men, on the other hand, tend not to be as talkative and tend to hold things in and may resent being prodded to be more expressive. As they say, it goes with the territory.

There are, of course, exceptions to both generalities. But from a psychological perspective, talking and communicating is healthier.

And then there are special needs listening. Many Parkinson's patients suffer from voice issues and vocal power and weak volume production. The voice can become gravely garbled to some extent and at low volume, making it difficult to understand what the patient is trying to communicate.

On top of this, vocal issues may be coupled with various levels of dementia. Asking a patient to repeat themselves or the thought just stated so you can hear it again and interpret to respond correctly may be impossible for them. If you don't pick it up the first time, you may have to say to the patient, "I didn't quite understand all you wanted to say, could you repeat that?" or "Is this what you wanted to say?" The patient can often indicate positive or negative and you can try again. But don't push. Take your time and keep it low-key, low pressure, and wait for a response. Patience here is called for and lots of it.

In extreme cases involving dementia, one has to again, use patience, and try to discern the wavelength the patient is on. But also, there are times this will not be possible. However, do not assume guilt for this. It is sometimes just the way it is.

Caring for One's Spouse

Perhaps the most difficult instance of caregiving is when one has to care for an ill or disabled spouse. Many various aspects are associated with this, and most are especially difficult but need to be addressed and will consider them head on.

To start with, the age of one's mate plays an important role in what the nature of the caregiving has to be. Naturally, the older the patient, the more difficulties there are likely to be.

We'll begin with the pain of memories when one looks back on the shared life together. Even if there are many good ones, one mourns for those days that are no more, remembering more happy, healthy times when life seemed more carefree with one's life ahead of them. And the longer one has been married, the more memories, thus the more bittersweet and at times painful those memories can become. But at the same time, paradoxically, the more blessed in their recall from a good life well shared.

Regardless of where one finds oneself at this point in a marriage, it is always better to say we have and had a good one. It is understood that life, being what it is, we will likely encounter difficulties as we move along through it into old age, which the Bible refers to as the "evil days" (no punches pulled here).

The one you're caring for may require help dressing, bathing, lavatory, getting in and out of bed and up from a chair, and perhaps some assistance eating, such as cutting food into smaller portions, etc. (which can engender some embarrassment to the one receiving care).

If you have the physical strength to do what may be required, you are fortunate, but if not, additional outside care may be needed. The installation of grab bars and a riser for the toilet seat makes things a lot easier and safer. Also falls can be a special hazard; therefore, try to assess and anticipate "trip spots" such as loss rugs, step ups or overs such as a threshold between rooms, even if very low. Slippery floors may require the patient wear skidproof shoes or socks. And if you must or prefer to use a second floor in your home, consider a stair lift if you can afford one, as well as a cane or walker for one-level management.

If a wheelchair should be necessary, you will need a ramp or lift to enter your home. In certain cases, financial assistance may be available to help with these installations.

You may want or need to consider some home care assistance as well—if for no other reason to free the caregiver (often the mate) to handle out of home tasks such as banking, food shopping, and other shopping in general—not to mention giving the caregiver a little needed break. As no matter how much you love someone, the task of caregiving is very wearing and taxing, and breaks are definitely needed for maintaining the well-being of the caregiver.

The Mental/Spiritual Side

Caregiving has other aspects besides the physical; some of which are most difficult to deal with and express.

The first area we will deal with is the area of sexuality. If you are still of an age where sexual relations are desired or were engaged in prior to illness, you may and are likely to find this a tough area to negotiate, and you may find it troubling that this can no longer be engaged in.

You may even find yourself beginning to fantasize being with someone else or a previous acquaintance or seek satisfaction elsewhere. We are and have been created as sexual beings, and it doesn't necessarily come with an On and Off switch. This is an area where Satan loves to hit you and can have a field day with you here. It is a psychologically dangerous area, and you must expect it and guard against it, as you will be especially vulnerable at this time. You will need God's special help here as well—and don't be afraid or hesitant to ask Him. And also, don't be embarrassed to bring it to Him as He was not embarrassed to create it.

All couples are different, and therefore, it holds in how they need to approach this most difficult and sensitive area. But discussions with each other in how to come to terms with this is a good and necessary thing. Men may find this more difficult to approach—women perhaps less so. But at any rate, look for openings where the subject can be eased into. A good opening line might be, "Honey, just want you to know I miss those times we made love, but I'm OK with that." A simple remark said with the right inflection can relieve lots of pressure on both sides and lets each party know that side of their relationship is still valued and missed. And it keeps one from feeling that they are no longer loved by the other.

And some other troubling thoughts you might find yourself having, for instance, "I wonder if I had married so and so if they would have turned out to be healthier" or "Maybe I should have married so and so." Thoughts like this can rush in like a flood and cause psychological embarrassment, particularly under extreme stress, but as a believer, you should realize the origin and source—the pit of hell. Satan knows where and when to attack us. It's not that we don't have our own failings, pretentions, and imaginings, but in a weakened state emotionally, they can run rampant and can be fueled by evil like a wildfire. So be sure to stay close to God during these times.

In life, we cannot prevent all illness, but we can learn to deal with it. Doing so will increase our spiritual strength in many ways—keeping in mind this life is preparing us for greater things to come and god uses all things to form us and prepare us in this regard. He says, "When you fall into various trials and temptations, count it all joy!" No, it is not fun when you are going through it, but there is a deeper purpose.

So while you must expect and guard against bad thoughts, the one thing not to do is to take on guilt. When God saved you, He already knew all about you and what you've done and thought and what you will do. We are all capable of some nefarious things when you come down to it, much as we hate to admit it. But instead of guilt, confront these thoughts and roar back against the evil forces that are trying to come against you. You know to whom you belong, and you need to rest in that day-to-day. And expect that God will help you in this area. And finally, realize that He created you too in His will and pleasure to love be loved and to be a blessing.

A Caregiver's Demeanor and Attitude

As has been said from the beginning of this book, caregiving is no easy task, but how it is administered is all important and has a lot to do with its effectiveness. In short, how it is received by the one being cared for. It helps first to perhaps get a better handle on the term *caregiving*. Maybe a better term would be "life assistance given with care." What a caregiver is really doing is helping their charge to keep going on with life in whatever state or disability they have.

Often the caregiver is so intent on providing the care, they overlook how the patient themselves feel as the care is being administered. Most tasks involved in doing this take more time—sometimes a lot more time—than under normal circumstances and capability of the patient. There is a tendency at time to try to rush, urge, or hurry the patient through them. This can make the patient feel anxious, tense, or afraid.

One of the emotions most common in caring for the Parkinson's, Alzheimer's, or elderly patient is fear and anxiousness. Hurrying a patient tends to make these emotions worse.

Male caregivers, especially spouses, tend to be offenders of this principle. The male tends to approach these situations in a business, no-nonsense-like manner. Efficiency and competent management of the situation is the goal or the objective as it is tied in with running the household as well. Pushing to keep things moving along seems to be the natural work mode. On one level, it makes sense, but on another it doesn't.

The other day, my lovely wife reminded me, "I just can't do the things needed as fast as you would like me to. I just can't go that fast."

And she was 100 percent right. In my zeal to get things done, I overlooked the true purpose of it all. I was not considering how she felt not being able to do all the things that had now become my responsibility. I was taken aback and hurt at first until God helped me realize that it was her feelings that counted, not my getting things done.

I further realized I had to employ much more patience and understanding and apply much more ingenuity and creativity to preserve our quality of life, which is the deeper objective of caregiving. In short, anything that tends to upset that has to be rethought or readjusted.

So once again, another point or area where God's input is vital. Yes, the body we have in this world will give out, but God is renewing the inner person who will someday receive a new permanent one. It is important to understand this truth, and in the meantime, always minister to the feelings of the inner person and the one you are caring for as they are as deeply loved by God and the one giving the care.

And finally, sometimes it is necessary to be abrupt or take charge in a dangerous situation such as an impending fall or touching a hot stove or the like. But even when that is necessary to employ, follow it with an apology or an explanation that you sensed danger and were trying to prevent injury. (A kiss followed by some ice cream can help here too!)

Caring for Someone with Mental Issues

Dementia presents another area of great difficulty. When someone does not perceive reality properly, it will seem like the person you know, have known, and love is not quite there anymore. I think it would be accurate to say, we'd rather deal and care for the physical side of things than the mental—and the reasons are obvious. Dealing with the physical can usually be handled a lot easier than the mental, and if you are handling this type of situation, you already know this.

While medical science is researching many diseases trying to find cures and management medications and treatments, what it has not had a lot of success in is the mental side of things. This just gives us an indication of how complex a creation we are. If you are dealing with someone with dementia, you now realize how much help, love, and support someone else you know needs—and that includes yourself in the caregiving role. Medical science would just love to find a cure for all illnesses, and if not that, an effective management so someone might return to or continue with normal living.

The very fact that people become sick causes much anger to be directed toward God. This is understandable and may cause some to be angry but may cause others to say or conclude there is no God. Extreme emotional pain can cause reactions such as this. Well, God handles your anger, but you must start to comprehend why this condition of "fallenness" and pain exists. In a book I've written called *Living in a Fallen World*, the issue of why this happened and what will, in time, happen next is dealt with. But the main thing to understand is God requires us to come to the conclusion that His character is the only way true life can exist. Through His leading us, we are brought to the point that we ask God to make us like Him and give us eternal life. It is referred to as being born again or saved through grace, or perhaps a better way to understand it is we are recreated—a new creature in His likeness. When that happens to an individual, we still continue in this life/world as it is, but we're different now—a new creation as God calls us, and this life then becomes a "school house" that prepares us for eternity to come.

It's not that continuing on is easy—no, sir—but through the eyes of faith, we see (and feel) there is a purpose to it, causing things we have to deal and cope with to take on new meaning and dimension. We start to overcome the negative with God's positive. We, in fact, war against the negative with God's positive. "The Spirit wars against the flesh [the worldly issues]" (Galatians 5:7).

We are, in fact, in a battle day-to-day to master the negative (with the help of His spirit) in this present life with these present bodies, and in so doing, we are termed overcomers. Yes, caregiving is a great challenge and responsibility in this regard, and if you are called to be one, you will require much godly wisdom in carrying out this assignment—or we may say a course God has laid out for you.

Many illnesses can produce dementia and mental misperceptions, and we will look at the matter more closely in subsequent chapters.

The Mind—Where Life's Biggest Battles Take Place

While we live and operate in a physical world, it is our thoughts and the working of our minds that determine our actions. A tasty example would be "I feel like having some ice cream." Now before you've had your first taste, it was the thought in your mind that came first and that resulted in the action which followed. This is a pleasant example—kind of like deciding what color your new car should be. We can cite many other such examples, and so can you.

However, there are those thoughts that are not so pleasant. Here is where conflict comes in and where the battles rage. While not all thoughts of conflict are bad—as this is part of problem solving—there are those thoughts that can rush in like a flood and play havoc with our emotional state. An example of this would be a recovering alcoholic having an urge to take the drink that they are not supposed to have. Or the smoker trying to quit cold turkey, wrestling with the urge to have a puff or two (of which there is no such thing in practical terms). These, of course, are bad enough. But the next level is the deep anxiety connected with dealing with serious caregiving problems.

A lot of these thoughts come under the heading of the what-ifs—the what if this happens or that happens. Some of these thoughts can be connected to problem solving, like anticipating and preventing falls or other hazards. These come under the heading of awareness suggesting appropriate action. But then there are the thoughts of doom or destruction—thoughts that don't lead to a positive action.

One of these is the constant anxiety of the day-to-day 24-7 dealing with caregiving a spouse, parent, or child. Frankly, there are not too many laughs involved here.

But let's consider a couple of thought battles that are real battles of conflict. A common one is a spouse battling whether to have an affair or not. Another would be deciding when to put a loved one in a nursing care home. I cite these two because I know many have these conflicts.

Most, if not all, affairs end badly, and if not badly, they end, sometimes by mutual agreement and sometimes by one or the other party. Affairs are seldom about companionship (although that could be the drive on senior level) but almost always about sex. I challenge anyone to dispute this.

The second big conflict—when to commit one to a home—can be related to the first (sorry to put it that bluntly) but can also just be a simple desire for freedom having been worn out by the world of 24-7 care. I submit if it is your mate at the root of this conflict, you've got a mighty big one to handle. If a parent a little less of one as sometimes an elderly parent will still have the parental instinct of wanting to make something better or less harsh for their offspring.

Either way, these are big battles waged in the mind, and there are no easy answers. But the answers one must seek is the wisdom, thoughts, and will of God. I submit once again that God's answers will bring you peace and the "wrong answers" will bring you even more agony and conflict in the mind. And along these lines, if you run a conflict answered wrongly out to its conclusion before any action has taken place, you'll come to the danger signs and barriers in the road. My advice—heed them.

Life is generally lived and worked out day-to-day, and it is a good way to approach these battles and conflicts.

Parkinson's and Its Special Needs

Parkinson's has sometimes been referred to as a "designer disease" because no two people seem to get it or exhibit its symptoms in quite the same way. It can manifest symptoms from quite mild to quite severe, and it is progressive. Parkinson's patients are sometimes told by a physician not to be overly concerned about having it as "no one has ever died from Parkinson's." While that may be true in the purely physical sense, it so greatly erodes the quality of life as it progresses that it is a kind of slow death, as one's abilities to do even simple things such as writing or signing one's name becomes an impossibility.

Diagnosing Parkinson's is different from most other illnesses as there is no blood test to determine or indicate its presence. Therefore, it is diagnosed or inferred based on symptoms, either individually or collectively. The common ones are a halting gait, sudden freezing of mobility (dyskinesia), loss of smell, memory problems (particularly short-term), dementia, hallucinations, tremors and difficulty controlling movement, diminished vocal and speech volume, frozen facial physiognomy (expressionless), and maintaining balance issues. And there can also be digestive problems as well since, basically, all bodily functions are affected and slowed down.

The cause of this condition is the diminished production of a brain chemical called dopamine—a neurotransmitter produced by the hypothalamus, an endocrine system gland, positioned at the base of the cerebral cortex an above the pituitary gland. With less dopamine than the brain requires, messages sent from the brain throughout the body are not as strong as they should be. It is this weakened transmitted signal that is causing the symptoms observed in Parkinson's. One can then say that the weaker the signals sent, weakness and control problems will be manifest in this disease.

To date, it is not known why the thalamus might not be producing enough dopamine, but it was discovered that the chemical dopamine could be replicated with a substance manufactured called carbidopa/levodopa in which this compound working together can often bring the patient to near normal capacity—but not always. A second substance acetyl choline and enzyme manufactured by the body from choline acts as a facilitator in receiving sent neuro messages from the brain. So nutritionally speaking, getting enough of this element helps on the other end of things to receive the weaker messages. Think of it as a bigger magnet or a ballplayer using a larger glove.

Besides the carbidopa/levodopa (medical name Sinemet), there are other drugs called agonists, which can be used separately or in conjunction with Sinemet and they help the Sinemet to be more effective. I won't list them here but sometimes in the early stages of Parkinson's, one of these alone or in combination can be effective in treatment, and often a physician will delay introducing Sinemet until absolutely necessary as it is the most effective med to date, and introducing it too soon will diminish its continued effectiveness over the long run. My wife who has Parkinson's was able to go well beyond twenty years on Ropinirole (Requipe)—an agonist—before taking Sinemet was necessary. Her case, for many years, remained mild, and only in the later stages was a stronger med necessary. But it must be stressed that each patient with Parkinson reacts and progresses differently, so there are no hard and fast rules, and it takes a very skilled neurologist to determine and manage, together with patient input, what will work.

For a Parkinson's patient then (as with anyone), good nutrition is important and is part of the treatment and therapy. While it is thought poor nutrition or missing elements from one's diet might have something to do with developing it—as might heredity—this as yet has not been conclusively established. Some researchers believe environmental pollution may be a causative factor. However, that too is not known. But from what we've seen in the curing of other diseases, it may take decades of research before a cure or cause is found. Some research of late has been looking into the function of the pituitary gland (the master gland), which is the manager of the endocrine system as perhaps not telling the thalamus to produce enough dopamine. No conclusions yet, but in research, you must turn over every stone.

In any case, as with age, Parkinson's is progressive and in time, symptoms tend to worsen requiring more medication in increased dosages, which brings us to how it is treated medically.

Treatment and Managing of Parkinson's

To begin with, like most patients and illnesses, treatment is an individual thing. However, with Parkinson's, which 1 percent of the population develops, can be even more difficult due to vast differences in patients. It helps if the neurologist treating the patient is integrative, in that all elements, are brought into play—medical, nutritional, physical, and spiritual (which is a good approach with any illness).

It was mentioned earlier that Parkinson's is a "designer disease" in that no two people seem to have the same mix of symptoms, although the symptoms do have a commonality in patients. Because of these patient differences and responses to treatment, neurologists often use the term trial and error in treating it. One reason for this is that there is, as yet, no definitive blood test that reveals how the endocrine system is managing the supply of dopamine to the brain or, for that matter, the presence of Parkinson's. The diagnosis itself relies on the outward observance of the common symptoms associated with it. The physician must ask the patient questions as to memory and observe the patient's reactions to certain aspects (e.g., balance, reflexes, strength, and flexibility as well as asking the patient how digestive, and elimination functions are working as well as sleep patterns). In this regard, the caregiver seeing the patient much more than the doctor can supply needed data on many day-to-day notes. This can be of great medical assistance. And it is also understood that medications are subject to change as the patient does.

Sometimes, patients become anxious or discouraged if the right meds and doses aren't determined at first try. It can often take a number of visits and tests to hit the right or best prescription. Patient counseling and understanding goes a long way to help with these fears and anxiety that accompany this illness. Joining a support group can be a real help here, not only for the patient, but the caregiver as well. Usually, the local rehab facilities know where these groups exist and how to contact one.

As important as medication(s) are the physical side, and if maintained to the patient's abilities, it contributes greatly to better functioning and well-being. If a patient has been physically fit throughout their life (walking, running, swimming, skiing, bike riding, golf, etc.), they will most likely want to remain so. However, for the patients (male or female) who are not, it may be difficult to bring them to a point where they will be more physical. The body, as has been said, was built to move and does not do well or as well when it doesn't. Truth is, being sedentary at any age is not good—even for the very young. No argument in medical science on this point. So whatever a patient can handle or accept (walking being one of the best), they should be encouraged to do so. It often helps if the caregiver will join in with the physical activity, such as walking together with the patient or working out with light weights together. Not surprisingly, both patient and caregiver will benefit themselves. Finally on this point, it's hard to exercise alone because, frankly, it's boring. But doing it with a companion can make all the difference. In the case of a married couple, many fine reminiscences have been shared on a good walk (with perhaps some ice cream afterward).

As PD progresses, there will be understandably less capacity for the physical, but whatever the patient can manage, again, should be encouraged. Exercise also releases something called endorphins in the brain, and these cause "mood upticks," which someone with a disability is always in need of. Regarding the physical though, balance can become a real inhibiting issue, and falls are the PD patients single most contributor to injuries as well as their greatest fear. Arranging a home environment as free of stumbling causing obstacles as possible is a good and necessary thing. However, a patient may lose their balance and spontaneously tilt and fall (usually backward) even though no contributing obstacles or hazards are present. When a patient reaches this point closer care and awareness on the part of the caregiver is a necessity. (My own wife has experienced a lot of these episodes which, in most cases, though not all unfortunately, I've been able to prevent or catch. These can happen without warning—and it is in caring for her that has inspired me to write this book.)

The Spiritual Side to Illness

This goes hand in hand with patient mood and outlook, which, as with any serious or long running illness, may not be good. One must realize (at some point in life's journey) that this present life (life experience) is temporary but has an important purpose which is to prepare us for eternal life and our relationship with God. While no one wants to be sick or debilitated in any way, it comes about due to the fallen nature and condition of the world. God though actually uses our difficulties to teach us many things. And it might be asked, "Who is being trained and prepared for this more, the person receiving care or the caregiver?" The answer is, and while we can't quantify it, both!

It's also been said that God often, perhaps most often, does not remove obstacles but rather tends to take us through them. And one might add, He's with us all the way—even when it doesn't seem like it. What results from this is a sweeter spirit and a much deeper awareness of how special and deeply loved we are by Him who made us. His purpose is that we come to that same deep love and value of Him and of one another. It is His will that no one be lost or discarded (keyword *lost*) and have that same deep longing—especially though not exclusively, for our mate.

Yes, it hurts to watch one's loved one struggle, but we know in whose hands they are, and He holds all the cards, so to speak. And while we long for all this to be over, we at the same time are given the vision (the divine imparted outlook) of what is to come when all creation is restored.

Parkinson's and Other Disabilities from the Patient's Point of View

Any debilitating illness or injury presents a loss for both patient and those around them—family, friends, and caregiver. We'll take a moment in this chapter to place oneself in the patient's shoes, as it were, to gain a perspective on what the patient is feeling and going through.

Consider for a moment something you really enjoy doing or participating in and now imagine never being able to do it again. Not pleasant, right? Well, that's what day-to-day is like for someone with a serious long-term disability. So much of what we do is so instinctive and natural, like walking, climbing stairs, using a knife and fork, etc., that we seldom give much thought to not being able to do those things.

There was a time in my own life where running up and down a flight of stairs two or three steps at a time was no problem. Today however, I'd be foolish to attempt it, and I'm not disabled. Having reached age eighty, I must accept the fact that I cannot do certain things that I used to. That fact hasn't changed my life much, but I cannot climb a ladder without discomfort and therefore am hampered doing certain outdoor house chores such has gutter cleaning. And if one particular chore is high enough and necessary enough, I must employ someone else to do it. While perhaps a little humbling and a little expensive (but better than falling off a ladder), it's not going to give me sleepless nights or is a game changer.

But now consider someone with a lifelong beautiful handwriting who now cannot sign their name or a birthday card for a loved one (as is the case with my wife). Something like that sounds so simple and easy yet is now not possible can really bring a patient's mood and psyche down. Yes, it might be one of degree, but points can be reached where the disability has become quality of life altering. Hard for a patient to stay up and optimistic, I think you'll agree.

So the job of a caregiver is not just to help physically but psychologically as well. It is important to always make the patient feel they are still a person and a valued and loved person at that. As said in the introduction, we enter this world needing lots of love and care, and we journey out for most of us the same way.

It's been said that life is to be enjoyed. That's certainly is as true as anything can be, but with a serious disability such as Parkinson's presents, as well as other diseases and disabilities, there is less of it one can enjoy. So a sad, remorseful, despondent, perhaps even suicidal patient is not unlikely to encounter.

And many times the patient in acquiring an illness or disability feels they have let others down—spouse, family, friends, or perhaps a business. Yes, perhaps certain illnesses are the fault of the patient's lifestyle and habits, dietary or otherwise, but in truth, there are many unknown causes and, even if known, may not have been known to the patient or in their purview or control, such as the air we breathe or suffering an accident in a public conveyance. Yet many times, the patient will feel responsible and will require much assurance to help them see they are not.

Decline through the aging process is something we will all experience and contend with and, in so knowing, be glad and ready to administer love and assurance that the best is yet to come. Yes, this is a statement of faith, but it can be most powerful and comforting getting one through the worst of difficulties.

Caregiving—The Larger Picture

"Looking out for one another."

"Am I my brother's keeper?"

"Who is my brother?"

These questions and issues all relate to the story (parable—meaning a teaching story) of the Good Samaritan. The point of the story is an individual injured and lying by the side of the road who is spotted by a traveler, a Samaritan, who comes to this individual's aid—got him medical attention, care, and lodging—which he paid for and thus enabling the injured man to recover.

As things turned out, the injured individual and the Samaritan were from two different regions that did not get along. One might say they were forms of enemies. And yet the Samaritan helped at his own inconvenience and expense. Why? He didn't have to, but why did he? The answer and the only answer was that he understood something very fundamental, and that is we are all connected. Well, if this is so (and it is), what connects us? The fact and truth is we are all brought into being by the one God—the great I Am—the Creator of all things whose character permeates all that's good and what he demands of us.

Some might argue, "No, we're brought into existence by the human sexual act and its resultant pregnancy." Really? If one believes that, one has overlooked or is ignorant of scripture that states, "I formed thee in thy mother's womb." One might also continue to add, "I created the human body capable of bearing life."

Once you see that truth, others immediately come into focus. The second great commandment states, "We are to love our neighbor as we do ourselves." And another more controversial command that "we are to love our enemies" And why love an enemy? So that they might come to know and love God and then to serve Him. In so doing and enemy may even come to be a trusted friend. This world is full of surprises.

We might ask, "Who taught the Samaritan all this?" The answer is we all possess a conscience, an inner voice (many terms for this). Some have even used the term inner knower. I personally like this term as it conveys the fact that we can know things from within without necessarily hearing it from an outside source first. It all points to the fact that God can transmit truth to our inner spiritual being which then can be made active in life's day-to-day events. Our free will comes into play when we decide to obey that inner voice leading.

If you have a receptive spirit, God will tell you things. "If any man lacks wisdom, let him ask and it shall be freely given" (James 1:5). In short if one wishes to know the truth, God will tell him. God loves to reveal Himself in truth.

A fine Christian author Watchman Nee wrote a book entitled *God Tells the Man Who Cares*. And one of the things God loves to tell and show us is how we are to love one another. Put another way, if God loves or cares about something, you should come to care about and love it too.

When we get to care for someone or are given the responsibility to do it, we are given the opportunity to fulfill a special part of that commandment. If you are caring for a spouse, this should not be hard to see. Or for that matter, anyone really close to you such as a parent or child. But caring for a stranger allows one to relate in ways that can be blessings on both sides.

And when you get down to it, race and color don't matter much either. What does matter is the inner person. Many have realized that once the inner person is known, race and color—in short appearances—are either insignificant or actually come to complement and coincide with the inner personality. This is a remarkable and important understanding to come to. Another way to think of it is if someone just saved your life, does it really matter what they look like?

Communication Difficulties

Communication is a vital human function. We communicate with one another and we must. However, sometimes this becomes difficult for two main reasons: one is physical, the other mental, and we will treat them separately.

We'll start with the physical. Any patient may have difficulty communicating vocally due to an injury or illness involving the vocal cords. However, with a Parkinson's patient or Alzheimer's patient, there is a deterioration of the ability to speak over time or, put another way, to energize the vocal cords. Because Parkinson's affects all bodily functions in some way, it is not surprising that the vocal cords would be one. But in order for the vocal cords to operate, they must be vibrated by air passing over them—in short breath power—provided by the diaphragm, the disc-shaped central torso muscle that divides the chest cavity from the abdominal cavity.

Usually when a Parkinson's patient has low energy or low volume speaking, it is not the lungs that are at fault but the muscle that powers the lungs, or breathing, that is at fault. Because Parkinson's disease produces an overall bodily weakness; it is no surprise the diaphragm would be affected.

Most of us never think of this muscle as there is no need to unless you are studying to be a singer or to play a wind musical instrument. So we can say, if you're breathing, this muscle is operating. However, if one is involved in the aforementioned musical studies, it is necessary to become aware of it and its function. In short, the diaphragm is the sound power, and when it is hindered, lungs and vocal cords are not receiving the energy support or "production" needed, and weak speech will be the result. There are exercises to strengthen it though and should be employed when this condition is recognized.

First though, the patient must be made aware of what's wrong and introduced to the diaphragm strengthening exercises, and there are some simple ones that can be effective. Having the patient breathe in and out while their hands are place against the waist will build this awareness. Breathing in (full breath) and holding it several seconds, then breathing out and holding that several seconds, hands still placed over top of the abdomen, will get the point across. Doing this two or three times a day will help strengthen this mechanism. Deep breathing is also good as it helps maintain lung capacity. One important point though. Often when you tell someone to take a deep breath, they will raise the shoulders as if it will draw more air in. This is wrong as it creates a reverse vacuum in the chest cavity, and short windedness results—just the opposite of what one is trying for. So keep the shoulders relaxed and in place and concentrate instead on the diaphragm.

Patients are also taught to forcefully say words—or shout—anything that reenforces *loud!* It also will be noticed in Parkinson's that the patient will trail off in volume. They may start a sentence or thought at one volume and then that drops off so that the listener may not be able to understand the complete meaning.

As a caregiver, it can become frustrating and patience-testing to keep asking the patient to repeat themselves. You may and likely will find the need to ask the patient to repeat themselves, and you need to be prepared for that. The patient may insist or infer the listener has a hearing problem. Spouses can have some difficulty here because there is less inhibition in making that comment. Keep in mind that someone who is speaking, hears their own voice from within, and it will sound louder to them than the listener hears it. Also the one speaking knows in their mind what they want to say, but the listener can only rely on the verbal sound. Thus, only when the patient keeps being asked to repeat themselves by outsiders or strangers is the patient likely to realize it is their speech problem and not the listener's.

On a personal note, I experienced this very thing with my own dear wife. As time and illness progressed, it became virtually impossible to carry on a normal conversation, except for short phrase sentences. Men are not generally known for being prolific talkers. I'm not one of these, and one of the saddest and most difficult things to cope with and bear was the loss of comfortable spontaneous conversation. Again, it is one of those things we just take for granted and never consider that it may not always be so. It is at these times we must look to and trust God and His promises that it won't always be like this.

It's been said we all have crosses (difficulties) to bear, and to quote our Lord, "In this life [world] you will have tribulation" (John 16:33). And have them you will.

Diminishing conversation is a big one. If you find yourself with this challenge, you will have to listen more closely and perhaps respond with creative one-liners to keep things on track. And don't hesitate to have your own hearing checked so that you're sure you pick up conversational sound and articulation at the best level possible.

Managing Medications

Often one of the caregiver's jobs is to set up meds and manage the times meds are to be administered. And part of this is to anticipate when a med prescription has to be filled. Some meds might have to be ordered by the pharmacy, and this could take a day or two. In realizing this, allowing for the fact that it might be necessary for the pharmacy to order, you should allow a minimum of four days' supply to cover this possibility. Also keep in mind meds cannot be ordered too far in advance, therefore check with the pharmacy on this. But in general, if you maintain a minimum four days' supply, you're safe. But also allow for the fact that when a med has to be renewed by the physician, take into account things could fall on a weekend (or if the doctor is on vacation) so authorization time may be increased beyond four days. Generally, if this happens and you're caught short, the pharmacy can advance you a small amount of the med to carry you through the med gap. The doctor's receptionist, if she can be reached, can usually do the same.

In managing meds, it is important to observe the reactions of the patient to them and note changes, problems, or irregularities. Parkinson's patients, reportedly up to 50 percent or more, will develop hallucinations and dementia. These can be troubling to both patient and caregiver. In communicating and responding to a patient, you will often have to field irrational questions or statements. This can be most difficult and troubling, particularly to a spouse. Often, the irrationality of questions and responses is actually the patients' difficulty in expressing their thoughts and not necessarily irrationality. This condition can vary from hour to hour and is believed to be related to the medications themselves. This is a classic catch-22 situation. You need the med, but the side effect is undesirable. In any event, try to remain calm and discerning and try to help the patient find the words to express thoughts or wishes. And again, much patience is called for in this regard.

Dementia and Hallucinations

Without a doubt, having dementia and hallucinations is the saddest and hardest aspect of Parkinson's or Alzheimer's disease to deal with because, though the individual suffering with it is physically present, the personage appears to be absent or distant. At least this is my opinion shared by many. I won't pull punches here. If this is what you are now contending with, you are in a whole new ballgame.

The mind is a mysterious thing, and no less mysterious is thought itself. We can't see it or touch it, yet all the issues of life proceed from thought. It is how we know we exist. Freud and Jung spent lifetimes studying it, and I dare say were perplexed by most of it. However, when the mind or thinking or perception become skewed, not so good things take place.

We'd love to know what causes this to happen so we could manage or control it. In Parkinson's, it is thought the meds themselves cause misperceptions (hallucinations) and mental scrambling, but until we know how to cure or stop this, we will contend with situations which can try one's emotions, patience, and energy.

If you are new to this situation, the following examples will give you a better idea of what the patient experiences. The fact is though, that 50 percent of Parkinson's patients will experience these symptoms and anomalies. Most of us are familiar with the individual in the desert dying of thirst and dehydration suddenly seeing before them an oasis containing water even though it is not there. However, to the individual, it is they literally see it. The old expression "don't believe everything you see (or hear)" would certainly apply. You *see*, but it's not the eyes that see but the brain that interprets the visual image recorded by *sight*.

Another example is dreaming when asleep. We've all had dreams that in the midst of seemed real until we awakened, and sometimes the dream actually lingered a few seconds, so that at the point of sleep and wakefulness is an in between state where our mind knows we are now awake, but for a few seconds, the dream is there as it fades. Some individuals can recall dreams in detail, even when fully awake. But the problem with Parkinson's or Alzheimer's the two states merge and the dream or hallucination becomes perceived reality.

Medications have been developed to help control this symptom, but they are not tolerable or suitable for everyone. But if the patient can tolerate them, they can be effective in whole or in part. However, it may be something that will have to be lived with as unpleasant as that sounds.

So then hallucinations involve seeing things that are not here in physical reality, and the other side of that is thoughts and perceptions not rooted in reality. Some of the typical things seen in patients are as follows. Short-term memory loss is a very common one—one that is perhaps the most often seen. A patient may ask, for example, "What day is it today?" only to ask the same question minutes later, be told again, only to ask it several times again. Some other typical ones are as follows: "Where are we going today?" "What's happening today?" "Who lives in this house?" "How long have we lived here?" When did we buy this house?" Even after a number of answers and/or explanations, the same series of questions may repeat themselves tomorrow or several hours later.

Here, I am speaking from personal experience, and I would wonder why I was emotionally and mentally exhausted by the end of the day. If you've ever wondered what's so hard about caregiving, this is it! This condition is described as dementia (short for diminished mental capacity) and can be present together with hallucinations making it, at times, hard to assess the patient's present state of awareness creating many difficulties in communication.

Other things to watch for are safety concerns. The patient may turn on the stove burners intending to cook something and forget they're on. Or they may place something flammable on the stove on top of a burner (such as a pizza box) creating a stovetop fire (which actually happened in our household). Or still, perhaps, flushing something not flushable down the toilet.

The list of these types of things can become quite extensive, but you must become aware of the potentials and be on guard. The patient does not intend to by irresponsible or unsafe; they are just in an unaware state.

Returning to hallucinations for a moment, there are some suggested ways to handle this with the patient and we'll look at some.

In listing these, however, I don't agree with all of them and as we go along, and I'll tell you why. The way generally suggested is to humor the patient. Example, the patient thinks they see a cat and comments on that, so you say, "Oh what color is it?" or "I like cats too." In either case, you are reinforcing unreality, and I personally disagree with this form of humoring. I'd rather say, "You know, I like cats too, but I don't think there is one there. Perhaps you see a shape that looks like one." Bringing the patient back to reality may, in the long run, be more helpful. You may have to be more patient, creative, and perceptive to do this, but I believe it is the better approach both for the patient and the caregiver (and again now you know why I'm tired by day's end).

It should be noted as well that the misperceptions state may come and go, and if you know the patient (as in the case of a spouse or child), you'll be able to tell when they are "here" and when not. You might also find it is timed to the medication dose and the time of day.

Hallucinations have another aspect though that can become a dangerous situation. If the patient owns firearms and thinks there is a nonexistent intruder, they may seek to take action against the phantom intruder, and I've heard of circumstances where police intervention was necessary to prevent tragedy and the confiscation of those firearms. It is obvious then that firearms and hallucinations don't mix.

Also, it must be determined if the patient is still perceptually fit to drive. Avoiding something in the road that is not there or running into something that is but not perceived can and has happened— usually before family and friends realize this is the case. While no one wants to confiscate the keys to a patient's car, sometimes for the safety of all, it must regrettably by done.

The deep sadness experienced in a spouse's decline from either Parkinson's or Alzheimer's is, as Nancy Reagan put it, "a long goodbye." Yes, no punches pulled here. But I hasten to add, in faith, on the other side, it will be "an eternal hello."

Maintaining One's Own Well-Being as a Caregiver

It almost goes without saying that you cannot help someone else if you are disabled. In short, you must maintain your own mental, physical, and spiritual state. When you have read and considered all in this book, you now understand the title.

I'll say frankly, one would love to flee, to escape the pain—the relentless day-to-day and all that goes with that. But that's how big difficulties and problems are. We just want desperately to get out from under. However, that's not why we are called to do certain things. Easy things don't teach much, and our life lessons go with us into eternity—even if our Bentley doesn't.

Through it all though, you must maintain your outlook and identity. Hobbies, interests, goals, shared or otherwise, are part of this and what you were created to be and do. This, of course, is different for each one of us, but you get the point.

However, you might now be thinking, "Where do I find the time for me in all this?" To answer that question, I'd like to share a great life lesson I learned a long time ago while a freshman in college. In the second semester of that first year, I was given the opportunity to pledge a fraternity—a music based one—and a good one. But I was also on scholarship, and it was needed in my case and thus important that I keep it. To do so required that I maintain a B-cumulative average, and I did have fears the time necessary to devote to pledging might be a threat to that. Nevertheless, I went ahead and pledged anyway and did everything my wits would allow to get everything done (including places to hide and study). To my amazement, in four years (eight semesters), the semester that I pledged was my highest grade average of the 8! Sounds impossible, but my transcript proves it, and there are reasons it turned out this way, and it's good for all of us to understand why.

Then how does one do this? It's been said if you want something done, give it to a busy person. Why is this so? It's because busy people know how to get things done because they have to. Too simple a concept? A simple demonstration of this can be seen in the restaurant business. My dad, who was a head chef, used to say, "You'll get a better meal and faster when the place is busy than when it's not. Why? Simple, the cooks, servers, stoves, grills, whatever, are going full steam to serve everyone, and well! You'll notice your food will probably arrive hotter as well. Being this busy forces one to think and organize quickly. It's a challenge, but when you absolutely must do something, you most always can.

One technique is to be more efficient. Some simple household examples are as follows, and I'm sure you can come up with many of your own. Our laundry room is in the basement, so when a wash is brought down, one is brought up that's been in the dryer. Another is don't go up and down the stairs empty-handed. Trips take time, so if something can be done in one trip, plan to do it that way (*caution*: in one's zeal to be efficient, don't sacrifice safety). Or it you are washing the car, hose off the mats at the same time. Or if you're stepping outside to deposit garbage, retrieve the mail on the way back in. The term for this is multitasking, but these little things do add up. Errands can be organized and handled in the same way. For example, if you're headed for the bank, combine that with the post office, getting gas, and perhaps some light shopping or picking up a prescription.

At first, you might have to think a lot to organize, but soon these combinations will be second nature, and you will find you've gotten more done and things will be in better order. And along the lines of order, try to establish a set place for everything. A lot of time is lost hunting for car keys, check book, reading glasses, bills, scissors, tape, glue, screwdriver, tissues, paper towels, etc.—anything you can think of. And declutter if you can. Clutter affects mood and efficiency, plus the house will always be presentable if unexpected guest(s) drop by.

In some cases, you may have to wait until your spouse or charge is asleep to have some free time. As everyone's situation is and can be different, this must be worked out individually. However, many a best seller has been written after hours, and many have been read the same way. Also, if you enjoy listening to music but do not want to disturb one's mate, headphones offer an answer. As a musician, I actually prefer the greater fidelity and special effect and presence using them.

To reiterate the point of this chapter, it is important to maintain one's own godly identity through the trials of caregiving. But in the midst of them, you might find an aspect of your identity you didn't know was there. This can be both positive and negative. But God often uses trials to clean house in our character. And it's good to remember the scripture, "I can do all things through Christ who strengthens me" (Philippians 4:13), and this one as well, "Our life (true identity) is hid in Christ" (Colossians 3:3). Many in the caregiving role have found they could do and handle that which they never thought they could.

Many a husband in having to handle most, if not all, household duties and functions has discovered how hard his wife worked all those years. And many a wife has discovered all the things her husband could do that now must be handled in other ways or by others. A good marriage is a partnership, and that takes in many things. Many a spouse has had to pitch in and do what the other always took care of.

While I'm a capable skilled handyman (but I'm not fond of plumbing issues) in most things, my wife never hesitated to do what might be considered a male purview. One day, years ago, I arrived home from work, and pulling in the driveway, I looked up to see my wife perched on the edge of the one-story roof section of our house, cleaning gutters! I never asked or suggested that she do this, but she took it upon herself to help out. And this was after working her own job in the dentistry field. Now that she's at age eighty and with

Parkinson's, one cannot imagine she could once do this—and do it carefree. But this is an example of crossing the lines in a partnership.

In the age to come, I'm sure we'll have a good time recalling things like this even though for now, no more gutter cleaning or sitting on roofs.

But to close this most important chapter, much help and grace is needed from God in order to carry out a caregiver's role and be able to remain a strong person with one's identity and inner being preserved. And a caregiver should never hesitate to ask God for this help—as he is the ultimate Caregiver.

Efficiency Tips

As this chapter is dealing with finding time for all that has to be fitted in daily and finding time for oneself too, here are some of the things that I have found to be time robbers in my own situation and some tips to solve this. I think you will find they are much the same for all caregivers.

1. Items. This is a big time robber (or waster, if you prefer) which is why I put it first: that is looking for lost or misplaced items. Among those are car keys, reading glasses, scissors, tape, glue(s), check book, recent bill(s), an article of clothing, tape measure, index cards, phone numbers, pens or pencils, writing pads, and blood tests and other medical information such as appointments.

    I'm sure you can come up with things of your own, but I've listed the everyday items that sometimes (too often) get misplaced. What I'll do now is take each item I've listed and tell you what we've done to solve it. But to start with, it means finding a place for these things and sticking to it.

    -   *Car keys.* We've hung hooks in the kitchen for not only the vehicles but the sheds and the lawn tractor. They can be decorative or simply nails in a board (but paint it a nice color).

    -   *Reading glasses.* Men, keep a pair in your shirt pocket at all times and one by the computer and the chair in your living room where you sit. (I even keep a pair in my trombone case.) Women, keep a pair in your purse as well as the other locations and perhaps one at bedside.

- *Scissors.* We've placed a small revolving caddy on the kitchen counter that holds a number of them in all needed sizes and types. It takes up little room and is always handy when most needed.
- *Tape.* Place a tape dispenser on the counter or island in your kitchen and perhaps one more elsewhere, perhaps at a laundry folding table or craft table—and keep it supplied.
- *Glues.* A small box holding all the types of glues you generally use can be tucked away with the pots and pans out of sight but handy.
- *Checkbook.* Keep in a drawer where you do the bills.
- *Incoming bills.* Open ASAP and write on the outside envelop amount due and due date. This will keep your bill paying timely and keep your credit score high!
- *Article of clothing.* If you intend to wear it the next day, locate it today and hang on hand where you dress or if a coat of jacket, where you keep outer garments. And if you can't find it, go on and pick something else until it turns up.
- *Tape measure.* A small on hand tool kit containing a tape measure, utility knife, several common screwdrivers, adjustable wrench, and small hammer for hanging pictures will take care of most small daily situations.
- *Stationary items.* You need a desk with drawers (where you write bills or where the computer is) and assign a drawer(s) for these. And don't forget rubber bands.
- *Medical and other important papers.* A small file box is the way to go.
- *Phone numbers.* A small indexed book works well, but we've supplemented that with a small index card box (our rolodex) for all those odd numbers seldom needed like an electrician or plumber.

The main thing is a consistent place for those common items you are always needing and misplacing.

2. The itinerary list. If you've been a caregiver for any length of time, you've discovered there is not enough time in the day it seems and the day zips by with, perhaps, little done except the bare necessities. What accounts for this and no, you are not losing your mind. Two things account for this condition: the one being the care that must be given the individual and the second is that simple things involving the one you're caring for just take longer—sometimes three to four times longer. So anywhere time can be saved or used better is important.

   As a help in this area, may I suggest an itinerary list made out the night before. This should include what you (and your charge) need to do and the order it must be done. A typical one from our household would look like this: (1) start today's laundry, (2) write bills that must go out today (3) mail at post office, (4) stop at bank to transfer funds into checking, (5) stop for gas in vehicle, (6) stop for milk, (7) morning nap for patient, (8) put wash in dryer and bring up yesterday's wash from dryer, (9) get take-out lunch, and (10) do a particular chore around the house.

   Your list may not have to be this elaborate, but I have found on certain days that have a lot packed into them, the list keeps everything focused and you don't miss appointments. I often jot down my list while we watch TV in the evening. It's easy to do and brings the patient into it as well as we consult as to what has to be on it.

   Index cards work well for these.

3. Food shopping list. This list can be done at the same time. In our situation, it is almost repeatable as we like the same things and generally follow the same eating pattern with diversity thrown in. Try not to make eating boring by not enough variation! And if you can't get out to shop, many food chains now deliver and will take your order over the phone.

4. Eating-out list. Once you discover what you like and what fits in with the budget, try, again to vary it. Don't eat the same thing every Wednesday, and a couple of times a month, make it a special one. And by special, I mean one that is beyond the daily allowance if you can manage that. If it should be that your charge can no longer manage eating out, shift to creative take-out.

5. Paying bills: Caregiving activities can sometimes be so consuming; other things can be forgotten about or missed. One of these is bill paying. Bills being paid late will affect you credit rating negatively, so you want to stay current. If you pay bills the old-fashioned way by writing checks and mailing them, note how they fall each month and how they group themselves. You'll notice that they do. I generally pay bills three times a month or, in other words, three groups. Some bills come quarterly and some each month. I generally have to write twelve a month—sometimes more. But doing them in groups does save time and keeps them current.

To sum things up, try to organize things so that you know where they are when needed. As stated earlier, hunting for things wastes an enormous amount of time and creates a lot of stress, which can be avoided. You may wonder how things can go "missing" in a house, particularly one you've lived in for years. But as you've no doubt discovered they can. And that goes for important papers as well. If you can't find last month's *This Old House* magazine is one thing, but when you need the ownership papers for a vehicle you are about to sell or trade in and you can't, that will raise blood pressure. So do everything you can to remain organized. It pays off.

Memories Pleasant and Otherwise

We all accumulate memories as we move on through life, and the longer we live, the more we collect. Some of these are pleasant to recall, and some are not. And scripture states there are seasons for things—a time to plant, a time to be born, a time to die, a time to mourn, a time to rejoice (Ecclesiastes 3:1–8).

In the latter seasons of life, when so much of what was easy, normal, and taken for granted is no longer available, memories are what we must then rely on. It's been said we only remember the good times. Perhaps so or perhaps it is the discipline of our choosing. However, whether caregiving for a spouse or as a professional, you will get to hear and share memories and recounting. And you may get to hear the same ones many times! But be a kind, patient, and understanding listener as these memories and stories are an integral part of the life you're helping.

It's been said, "Be kind to everyone on the way up as you will meet them all on the way down." Relating this to memories, you will likely have many of the same—you just haven't gotten there yet. But when you do or are approaching that point, you might then recall your mom and dad or relatives telling the stories of what they did in life or what happened to them going through it.

I recall my Polish grandmother talking about relatives she left in Poland and the Ukraine and tearing up each time she recalled getting a letter from them recounting the suffering they encountered under the Communists. Though I never actually discussed these with her, I imagine she felt both guilt and sadness, as well as relief and gratitude that she and her husband and children were able to come to America. But her sadness did not stop there as during her life, she lost her husband and two of her three daughters, one of whom was my mom.

Sometimes, we just scratch heads or wring our hands in perplexity and cry out *why*? Yes, there are questions in life we can't answer. It's not that they don't have answers; we just don't know the answers. However, what or rather whom we should first seek to know is the One who knows the answers to all of life's issues and that is God Himself.

There is the biblical story of the Lord being summoned to heal a very sick child. But by the time the Lord arrived, the child had died, and the parents were in grief. "If only you had come sooner," they cried. The Lord replied that the child was not dead but asleep and that the event was not meant for evil but for good, and the child was promptly healed and restored to health. What then do we take away from this? It is that God is sovereign over life and death and that He always has the last word and purposes to everything.

If your spouse, child, or charge is near the end of their time and loss is imminent, you will have then the life memories until the restoration and the reuniting. It's been said that our memories keep a loved one alive in our hearts. That is fine and beautiful, but it is God who keeps the records of lives, and as Jesus once said to a group of "misunderstanders" that the Moses whom they revered was not dead even though his life passed from their presence, and to put it in the Lord's words, God is the God of the living and therefore (Moses now being with God) Moses is not dead.

In closing this chapter, God has made it clear that He is the life, the way, and the hope. And that life resides in Him and though our memories may be sad and painful, we can trust God who promises a reuniting, and though we sorrow, it is not without hope. And God would like this to be understood and hung on to in faith.

The "Grouchy" Patient

Some people (and patients are people after all) seem to have sunny dispositions despite their illness or difficulties—and some do not. Some may have dispositions that border on the terrible or just plain awful. In short, there is a big range. What accounts for this? We'll take a look at some reasons. And if you are fortunate enough to be assigned to someone who is sunny or pleasant, count yourself lucky and blessed as this is often not the case.

We all come with a past, and the longer one lives, the longer the past. What fills our past has a lot to do with our state of mind in the present. Most people start out in life with hopes, expectations, and ambitions. As part of this, we have an expectation of what we'd like our lives to be or just life in general. And as we go along, reality has a way of shaping what we come to expect from life.

It's been said life is full of disappointments. We come up against this all the time, and how we handle life has a lot to do with our disappointments and outlook. It's also been said that the face one has at age fifty is the face one deserves. We'll let the reader apply what's appropriate in this area. But we will deal with several areas that shape our state of mind and therefore our disposition—pain, remorse, self-piety, regret, satisfaction/wisdom.

1. Pain. A person in strong-enough pain is not likely to be too sunny. This speaks for itself. And yet there are those who manage to rise above whatever it is and still project a decent disposition. But if not, the caregiver should not expect a whole lot from a patient in severe pain. But if sunshine still prevails, it is, understandably, a rarity. Akin to this condition is paralysis. Some individuals confined to

a wheelchair or paraplegic have still managed to project a positive image. Two notable examples are Jonnie Erickson Toda and Charles Krauthammer. Their view of life, though intensely real and acknowledged, nevertheless did not prevent them from moving forward successfully in life to the shame of many who do not have their impediments.

2. Self-pity. Often, this attitude takes over a patient's outlook faced with serious, life-changing obstacles. A caregiver can help by learning of and reminding the patient of the good and positive things they've achieved in their lives. This is particularly important if the patient has no reasonable hope of recovery or reversal of their situation. In this state, a patient may remark and think, "Well, what have I achieved in life. I'm not famous or anything." Well, to begin with (and we all have to be reminded of this from time to time), becoming famous is not a goal. It is a result, and it is few that achieve wide name recognition. Better to be known for being a kind, helpful, and loving person who is in turn loved. And even if the patient has achieved some fame or recognition, the previous statement holds true, nevertheless.

3. Remorse. This is primarily a feeling of sadness in the things lost or not being able to be done anymore. This is most acute in the patient who has lost a child or a mate. Obviously, these cannot be replaced or restored here (although God could do it if it suited his will or purpose). In a case like this, the caregiver can remind the patient of the promises and assurance God has given us in His word that there will be a complete restoration ahead on a new heaven and earth (a restored one of perfection) for those that believe in His Son Jesus Christ. This becomes part of the blessed hope, and it's not just for a patient but for all who believe.

4. Regret. A feeling of deep remorse or anguish over things done that one wishes could be undone or things not done that should have been. When you analyze this point, most of this involves relationships with others, and you can fill

in the blanks. No need to spell these out as the main ones are understood by anyone who has lived a while. Along these lines, do not hesitate to tell those who matter to you that you love them, and don't let rifts between those you love go unresolved.

5.   Ambitions unfulfilled. We all have (or will have) hopes and ambitions we never get to fulfil or complete in this life. We just run out of runway, so to speak. But when you think about it, isn't that what eternity is for? We, being made in God's image, who loves to create, we have that same built in urge which doesn't go away. Looking at this another way, if you were an individual who had acquired and done everything you could think or hope for, then what thumb-twiddling time! We reflect our Creator in that we want to do, create, accomplish, go, see, and experience. All of us someday will reach the point of inability to do these further—whatever that was. Still, it is not the end of the story. But one who only sees the dismal side of their condition or restriction as a patient will not be a happy camper.

On a humorous note, there's the story of the politician, after losing the election, was overheard to remark, "And I was going to have a dark-blue limo!" One could call this a misdirected priority or remorse, but it shows something else. We as human beings are not perfect, and we eventually have, at least, some remorse and regrets. But if we have, with God's help, attempted to live life well and do and become where our gifts were directing us, we will acquire *wisdom* and *godly satisfaction*. These are great sustainers because we now see and understand two things. We have the acquisition of things accomplished and the understanding this drive will always be our nature and will be our nature in eternity. "My gifts are not refundable," saithe the Lord. The more we understand and see this point, the more we will be at peace and the more we can help our patients to see it too.

Yes, there is always the bucket list, but when you have forever to do all that's right and of good report and with those you love, you have godly contentment, and that, as God's Word says, is great gain.

The "Grouchy" Caregiver

Face it! Some days we just get out of the wrong side of the bed. And if you are a caregiver and your day began like that, you are going to have a tough day ahead. We're all human, and we can't all be at our sunny best 100 percent of the time. But in any job where you have to face or deal with the public or caregiving, it is important to learn the term "in spite of."

Two things! We have to try not to bring the "home to the job" or "the job to the home." Having said that, neither is easy. But then, we're not talking about being 100 percent perfect. Rather, we're saying be alert to the fact that you might not be at your best on a given day or situation. This can affect the one you're caring for, particularly in a spousal setting.

There are ways though that you can let the one you're caring for know that you yourself may be in need of TLC or understanding at the least. Leaving home that morning, having a sick child or a returned bill, car breakdown, your tree falling into the neighbor's yard and into their swimming pool taking out the perimeter fence in the process. You get the point. Stressful life events can easily be brought to the job, and if your job is caring for a loved one in your home, well, again you get the point.

The first thing to realize is make sure there is no immediate danger and then tell yourself, most everything gets resolved in time. I can't tell you how many dents, scratches, and rust in previously owned cars that I used to agonize over that now I don't even own— what a waste of time and energy that was! But nevertheless, patience and realistic thinking is called for in these situations.

On the other side of things, your patient may be having a bad day thereby stressing you. If it's not your spouse, at least you get to leave and go home at some point (so you can look at your tree in the neighbor's swimming pool—otherwise known as "bad day at Black Rock") and hopefully get to unwind. If it is your spouse or family member, you have no choice but to ride things out.

In that regard (it's been said nobody loves a grouch, except perhaps on Sesame Street), look for and draw on things that you know or at least were pleasant in the past. As a professional leaving for home, you may have to say to yourself, "I'll take the whole family out for a nice dinner, even if just at McDonald's." Or if a spouse, do the same if your patient is ambulatory. You can watch the DVD you like while you have some ice cream. (Ice cream is known to have many therapeutic properties.)

One thing that can ruin a day is dealing with *messes*, *spills*, and *accidents*. These will happen from time to time so be prepared. They may be falls, spilling drinks, or bathroom incontinence issues and accidents. These are upsetting to the patient and often occur later in the day when the patient is tiring. When they do occur, try not to show anger or annoyance; just deal with it as the patient is already aware and embarrassed and stressed and if not (due to dementia), it would be of no use to berate the patient. Not to put a downer note on it, but remember, someday it could be you in the same circumstance of life.

When things like this happen, one must think and say, "This too shall pass" and "We'll get through this together," and with God's help, you will.

The Dreaded "A" Word

A certain percentage of elderly patients will experience this dreaded ailment—particularly though not exclusively, those with Parkinson's disease. What makes this ailment so dreaded and sad is the loss of the person to themselves and their mate as well as family and friends. While we don't know exactly what a patient may experience in their consciousness or subconscious, the real or outside world can become strange and unfamiliar to them. This can include environment (home, neighborhood) and those they know well like a mate or family. You begin to see then why it is so upsetting and tragic.

You may think the patient can be talked back to reality, but as this disease progresses, they cannot. As a mate or caregiver, you must realize that and meet the patient where they are at the moment. During rational moments (an Alzheimer's patient can be rational at times and the percentage will vary from patient to patient), discuss, interact, and broach all subjects and items appropriate, but in those other moments, flow with the patient's perceptions and try to fit an appropriate response. This is not always easy, but you'll get better at this the more you do it. However, Alzheimer's patients tend to exhibit a lot of fear and anxiety, so go easy. Don't strongly insist they do or see something in a certain way, but gently key off what you hear and sense.

While there are new meds to ease the effect of this disease, patients do not recover from it but progresses to a terminal state. If you are the patient's mate or child, this is most disturbing and upsetting—no getting around it. You will need God's help, support, and comfort more than ever.

Caregivers often ask what the difference between Parkinson's and Alzheimer's is as so many of the mental aspects are the same.

While there is a blood test for Alzheimer's, there is not one, as yet, for Parkinson's, one would have to infer a difference by degree of patient mental disability. Technically though, Parkinson's condition is that the brain is not receiving enough dopamine—a neurotransmitter, whereas Alzheimer's is a plaque buildup in the brain that essentially starts blocking and inhibiting function, and to date, it is not known why either condition develops.

Losing a mate is one on the deep sufferings of life and many of the common platitudes won't fly right now. "Well, you've had a long life together" or "You've enjoyed such happy years together" might earn you a harsh, well-deserved response. Rather, we are to rejoice with those who rejoice and grieve with those who grieve. Best to leave it there and let God do the deep comforting.

At a time like this, you may be plagued with regrets. "I should have done that" or "We should have done that when we had the chance" or "I shouldn't have said that back then." Plus, it is extremely painful to watch someone you love suffer. Even the good memories can be painful at this time, as one longs for those better days.

I'll share a personal story from my past involving my widowed mother and the time in my life when I became engaged. My dad died several years earlier and left my mom a widow with myself as the oldest and three minor children. Plus there were financial difficulties that went along with this period, which included finishing a house my dad and I started to build—one that would replace the old one on the same property. A couple of years later, my mom met a widower, and a serious relationship developed along with a marriage proposal. However, my mom was diagnosed with ovarian cancer and became quite ill. On top of that, her intended disappeared suddenly, and it was obvious he didn't want to go through losing another mate. One can easily imagine the difficulties and complications that arose as a result.

At the time, I deeply resented the fact that he left this way and part of me still does. However, I also understand the pain and distress he must have felt. Dealing with my own wife in the latter stages of a serious disease, I don't think I can now judge him as harshly as I once did—at least in regard to his apparent emotional turmoil.

But now, enter the word *commitment*. If you vow and commit to someone, that should and must mean something. We all hope and wish for the best of happiness from our marriages and relationships, but we do not have guarantees in this life and world as it is.

Commitment then is a conscious decision of one's will and not necessarily of one's emotions. The emotions often say, "Run the other way," "Let me out of here," or "I didn't sign on for this." We are always warned not to make decisions based solely on emotions. But emotions can be and often are, so strong, it's hard not to. Before we throw the baby out with the bath water, we need to recognize their place in heightening the joy, meaning, and depth of experience. It is our wills that are supposed to control our emotions. But the generic societal world view tends to be the opposite, and living in this environment daily, we often come to think of emotion being what rules our actions. or should be the norm—a spiritual fallacy for sure.

However, before you consider bolting or a retreat, consider what that would mean down the line. Suppose you did flee the coop only to meet your loved one in eternity and how you would answer their question, "Why did you leave me when I needed you most?" I strongly suspect there would be a lot of hemming and hawing in a most embarrassed sheepish way—and well deserved. No, hard things are not easy, and it takes a lot of spiritual maturity to handle them. Plus, if you have children or other relatives and friends as well who were trusting and expecting a follow through or commitment, what would be your reason and response to them?

In short, in situations like this, you are the man or woman of the hour, and you have been placed—like it or not—in the front-row seat to manage and oversee this life development. Sorry for the lecture, but it is hoped you will come to see and say, "Thanks, I needed that slap upside the head!"

When it comes down to it, most life situations can be best understood and managed by reversing the circumstances. All one needs to do is ask, "What if this illness/difficulty were happening to me?" What would I be needing and hoping for? A faithful companion would, I'm sure, top the list.

It's been said if you depend solely on people or someone, you'll always be disappointed as they will always come up short. Perhaps so, but with God's help, *you* don't have to be a disappointment. Character matters, and it is in this extreme testing that reveals what we're made of. God says we are being refined as pure gold in fire. And he says He will turn up the heat and closely watch. Well, friend, this extreme testing of life is the heat.

Depression and Suicide

Once again, we tackle a very difficult subject, and as a caregiver, you need to know about it.

To begin with, even a mentally healthy person can suffer a period of depression when one becomes down due to some life circumstance. This could be physical in nature or mental due to family or job stress, lack of sleep, or perhaps poor diet or a strained relationship or disappointment about something in life's on goings such as losing a bid on a desired house or property. We can cite many more of these, but you see the point.

Usually though, once the situation becomes resolved in some way, the depression lifts—at least in time. And there are things one can do and concentrate on to resolve depression. One of these—and a good one—is having something to look forward to. This could be anything from a trip to a purchase of a long-desired item. The key here is feeling life is worth living and looking forward to.

However, given a severe long-lasting depression, this can change one's outlook, and life can appear to the patient as not worth living. You may hear someone say in this state, "I have nothing to live for." If a patient's depression is that serious and they start saying things along this line, the caregiver needs to be alerted to the possibility that the patient may seek to end their life.

If this becomes the case, why suicide? What does ending one's life have to offer? In the purest immediate sense, it is escape, escape from pain—physical or emotional that the patient no longer feels they can bear. The individual does not see life getting any better and sees suicide as the only alternative. A patient who has lost a mate may view suicide as a means of joining their departed loved one perhaps sooner than natural events would allow. Yes, there is this spiritual side to it, but most religious beliefs do not sanction suicide or approve of what should be God's prerogative or call regarding when a person's life should end.

As a Christian, we believe God orders our life paths and has a course laid out for us. To end it on our terms dishonors God's plan, wisdom, and purpose. Even insurance companies will not honor a policy activated by suicide, unless a time clause is specified.

But back to how a patient may look at things. Given strong enough physical or emotional pain, the patient's will to carry on may be just in a collapsed state. In this condition, the patient needs encouragement and purpose, and family members can help in this regard as can friends. Physical pain can be managed, but emotional pain is not so easy.

If the patient is ambulatory, or mobile, joining or being taken to a support group can be a big help. Being amongst those suffering from the same things and can commiserate and share life's events can help the patient see that others are in the same boat. This can often ease the feeling of "there's nothing here for me anymore." It gets the focus off oneself alone and puts it on others. Comforting another often brings comfort to one's self as well.

Input from clergy can be a very important antidote to this extreme fatalistic depression. Seeing things beyond oneself can often bring one around. It is something else to try, with the understanding that it can antagonize the patient if they have an antireligious attitude. One must know something about the patient's view of religion before suggesting the patient talk to clergy. Spiritual matters should, one would think, be a positive thing, but for some individuals, it isn't.

As a caregiver, one of your jobs is to be a watch dog for signs or things might be heading in the wrong direction psychologically, mentally, or emotionally. You often hear family and friends say about a suicide, "I never saw it coming" or "I just misread the signs" or "I knew they were depressed, but I never thought it was that serious." Sometimes we're just afraid to acknowledge the signs that are there. Misreading signs is sometimes a matter of ignoring them hoping they will go away. Yes, encouragement always—and when appropriate—are the proper prescribed "mood medications" as these can help restore the patient's outlook. But job one is to recognize and evaluate the signs.

There is a saying in Native American culture that goes, "Let me not judge another until I have walked in their moccasins for many moons." This can apply to many things, but in all of them, we are to step inside another's circumstance and ask how would I be likely to feel if that were me? *Caution*: we are not to become depressed ourselves in doing this, but it is a tool in patient care. At the same time though, you are often the first line of defense. But be aware also, you might not have many moons to react and alert those who can intervene and stop a potential tragedy. In your conversations with the patient, observe mood and/or changes therein and gently probe their outlook. If they seem withdrawn, suddenly quiet, or expressing a disinterested attitude in general, these are some common warning signs.

Caution: If the patient possesses the means and if you have *any* doubts or suspicions of patient suicide intention, don't hesitate but call 911 for intervention. You likely will have saved a life.

Having said all these things, it should be understood that we are not talking about end-of-life hospice in which, at this point, the patient wishes to and is prepared to depart.

Obviously though, a patient who can physically live on but wishes not to and may have already made attempts is the subject of this chapter.

And be careful how you phrase things to the patient. Saying "You know you have a lot to live for" may be true from your perspective but not the patient's, even though in the objective sense, it is true. You instead might say in reminding the patient, "You are loved by those who would miss you, myself included."

There is a railroad story that demonstrates many of these truths, and it goes. A young railroad worker new to the job was being trained for a station trackside position and was being verbally tested. The question he was given was this: suppose the board indicator should indicate there were two trains approaching each other on the same track—what would you do? The worker replied, "I'd make sure the signals were operating properly." The supervisor than countered with, "Suppose there was a power failure, and they weren't working?" The worker then replied, "I'd throw a switch and divert one train to a siding." The supervisor countered, "Well, suppose it was winter, and a storm froze the switch?" The worker replied, "I'd build a fire on the track." The supervisor countered with, "Suppose it started to pour rain, and all the fire material was wet." The worker responded, "I'd grab my lantern and run down the track and try to warn one of the trains." The supervisor countered again with, "Well, suppose you had no lantern oil or no matches." The worker paused and thought for a moment and said, "I'd run into town." The supervisor, surprised and taken aback, asked, "Why would you do that?" The worker replied, "I'd wake the town and tell them to come out and see the best train wreck they'd ever likely see!"

Yes, it's possible that despite everyone's best efforts, the worst could happen. We would hope not, but at least you would know you did your best. In the final analysis, the patient, like all of us, is responsible, and we must let God in his mercy be the Judge.

By way of an addendum to this chapter is the business of the wreckage left behind for those who are left after a suicide. It isn't just the loss of the person themselves but all the emotional damage for those who must deal with the aftermath. The first and most obvious is a loving mate and all the questions that remain and that is followed by family and friends. But often overlooked is the first person on the scene who discovers the body. This is not always the mate, but could be a child, relative, or friend. All of this leaves scars that can remain, often forever. One wonders whether the one who takes their life ever considers the aftermath? Perhaps, by the time one decides to check out of this life, the decision overrules everything else. This is one of the saddest parts of suicide as there is an element of selfishness in depriving your loved ones of your presence before it is your time. Many a note has been left expressing remorse for what they are about to do and the acknowledgement that they know it will be painful for those left and that they love (whomever). As you can see, there is a conflict here. There are many conflicts in life and in living, and this is perhaps the greatest—or at least one of them. The decision to stay or go? It can be argued that when the decision to take one's own life has been reached, a form of insanity has set in.

We will leave things at this point except to say, those left need much support, comfort, and understanding as there are lifelong questions that will constantly be wrestled with.

The Power of Music

"Music hath charms to sooth the savage beast" (William Congreve). We've all run across this saying, but is it really true? Yes, and a lot more. Music is the greatest mood enhancer there is, and we can and should use it in caregiving.

You can actually study music therapy as a branch of medicine; it is that effective in treating the psyche. There are reasons it is, and because it is my profession and area of expertise, perhaps I can save you some time and money.

We take it for granted and are not surprised when we find music is everywhere—stores, restaurants, airports, waiting rooms, gyms, etc. And don't overlook music's function in cinema as background to all types of scenes and emotions.

The reason is simple. The right kind of music can promote the mood and atmosphere we want the occupants to have. Studies have been done to show certain kinds of music can promote spending while shopping, which explains one place where music generally permeates. We are all familiar with stores playing Christmas music at that time of year, and it most definitely creates the mood for Christmas shopping. Music is atmospheric!

Music is comprised of three elements: melody, harmony, and rhythm. The melody is the tune, the harmony colors it, and rhythms are the propelling energy. The three in combination are equally important as the sum is greater than the parts, so to speak. Instrumentation are the devices that bring it to life, and that includes the voice as well. These elements combined in the right way can promote a good feeling or mood as well as stimulate physical movement. Music though can do the opposite as well. The next time you watch a movie, note the music as it relates to the storyline. What will the music be like in an action scene, a love scene, horror scene, and so on—different certainly. You'll note the music is distinctive in all of them. And you'll note also, music can telegraph what's about to happen.

Now in caregiving, we want to create a happy, relaxed, upbeat mood—one that will encourage and facilitate the sense of movement. As we know, music can vicariously be transmitted to muscle sense and memory, which is why music makes us want to dance. Remembering what the different elements are and what they do, the melodies should be clear, beautiful, uplifting, and the harmonies should complement that—no dark somber chords and heaviness. And the rhythm light, perky, and mildly energetic. An endless amount of music can be found or created using the elements this way. But if we were to give a name to this or categorize it, it would be light jazz, Latin or Latin jazz, such as the bossa nova. The selection "Girl from Ipanema" would be a good example. Light instrumentation works well too—piano, guitar, vibes, light percussion (drums) of all types and related Latin instruments. By the way, you'll note this music type is well suited to dining, as again it promotes a good, pleasant atmosphere.

Sometimes music cynics might refer to this as elevator music. But forgetting the cynics or musical snobs, it is effective for these purposes. In caregiving, you want to promote good mood and atmosphere. Do so if the patient doesn't object, but keep the volume down and listenable. Also learn and use the patients' music collection, if they have one and learn their favorites, many an interesting conversation has developed over music.

The Self-Preservation Instinct

Sometimes referred to as the survival instinct, it is something all humans are born with. It is the instinct that denotes danger and things harmful to one's safety and well-being, both physically and psychologically. It is that sense that says, "Run the other way" or "Don't go there" or "Don't eat that."

The role of caregiver can be one of those things that can make one want to run the other way and therefore can set up a real conflict in the caregiver. Elaborating further, watching one who is not doing well in recovery can be very stressful, particularly if it is a spouse or child but not exclusively so. On the one hand, part of you wants out but on the other, love compels you to stay. It is a conflict every serious, long-term caregiver becomes acquainted with.

Getting some time off, even for a couple of hours, support groups, friends, family, and church can be a great help, and also the awareness that something much better ultimately lies ahead for all who are rightly related to God.

Still though, serious caregiving is very painful and stressful and will tax the self-preservation instinct. But before you run the other way, halt, and ask yourself, "If I did remove myself from my loved one, have I really solved anything?"

I submit you would find you have taken even more pain and regret on yourself.

So instead, don't run, but stop, think, and pray!

Eating Disorders and Nutrition

Eating disorders fall into three main categories: eating too much, eating too little, and eating the wrong things. These can be applied to anyone, but disabled patients often have special needs and/or restrictions in this area, and we will discuss them.

Food intake is basic to life and good health. Notwithstanding the debates one hears about what foods are good or bad, food itself falls into several main categories: protein, fat, and carbohydrates. So no matter how you look at it, you're talking about meats, dairy, and fruits and vegetables (with some whole grain breads and pasta thrown in). And in general, you can't go wrong with a balanced varied diet consisting of those main food groups.

But before we get specific concerning them, we need to look at eating disorders first, as often, patients will have one or more of the following three, and therefore, caregivers will be contending with them.

1. Eating too much. Eating too much results in obesity, and this added weight to a patient makes physical movement more difficult as well a healing. The reasons why someone eats too much generally fall into several categories that can come under the umbrella of easing depression. The expression "comfort food" is a good one because the patient is eating to soothe their hurts emotionally and may not even realize this is what and why they are doing it. This is hard to deal with because it is a dependent addiction (yes, food can be an addiction), but it rarely gets called that. But a diabetic condition may too create a craving for food because of low energy and other related symptoms, so it is important to determine whether the patient is or is not one.

So if the patient is eating because they feel good when consuming favorite foods or just that it tastes good, it may be difficult to change the habit. But emotional support and counseling, along with better nutrition, can start to change things.

2. Not eating enough. The opposite can also be true with depression—losing interest in food or eating. The patient may be in a state of not caring about life or themselves, and food just does not interest them, or it loses its appeal. Also, patients who, because of their ambulatory state, are not or cannot get much physical activity, the hunger craving may be greatly reduced. However, in either state, not taking in enough nourishment works against the patient's recovery or day-to-day health. It is important then to determine the cause and try to make changes in the patient's outlook and exercise—to the extent possible.

3. Eating the wrong foods. And what are the wrong foods? There is a well-known expression among nutritionists which goes, "If man makes it, don't eat it!" Most of us like our ice cream, cookies, shakes, soda, or candy. I excluded chocolate because as of late, good benefits have been discovered in dark chocolate—just don't eat a whole bar at once. OK, well, occasionally is all right with the other stuff as we are not monastic beings (at least most of us). However, when the patient is craving ice cream mostly and other sweets and turns their nose up at real food, there's trouble brewing for two reasons: sugar and lack of nutrients.

More and more in the medical community, it is thought that refined sugar is a real culprit in good nutrition and good health. The reason is it causes inflammation to various areas of the body and is believed to be, perhaps, the main culprit in serious diseases like cancer, arthritis, heart disease, and others. There are chemical and biological indicators for this, and we won't go into chemistry here, but if the expression "you are what you eat" (and I will add, what you don't eat) holds true, then we all need to look at and understand as much about nutrition as we can. Unfortunately, most individuals don't know enough or anything at all and make the mistake of eating just for caloric satisfaction or 'til full and thus the term empty calories. Even doctors themselves do not receive enough nutritional training if any at all. It is rare to find a physician that counsels a patient on a dietary direction they should go. (And in fairness, many patients ignore dietary admonitions as well.)

But back to the difficult eater. In patients, especially the elderly, there is a tendency to like to eat sweets because they are pleasant tasting, and with diminishing taste due to age, this is understandable. Real foods that are pleasant tasting and easy to eat are seasoned chop meat, sweet potatoes (mashed), corn, whole wheat pastas (small size), apple sauce, mashed bananas (with wheat germ mixed in—even in ice cream). These foods mimic sweetness but are good for one. Ice cream is acceptable as it is a source of calcium.

Back to sugar for a moment. Products that are known to be harmful, like cigarettes, now come with a warning label. It is not a big stretch—if the thoughts about sugar hold true—sugar having a warning label as well. Refined sugar and certain food sugars, as said earlier, cause inflammation in the body and suppress the immune system. This, combined with stress (and who doesn't have that), causes the body to produce cortisol, which then causes the body to store unwanted fat. Stress alone can do this but combined with sweets and you have a formula for packing on the pounds. And something additional happens in that sweets produce their own craving addiction.

Manufactured sweets are not a natural food but have become part of our society and culture and so are considered OK—even celebratory (the wedding cake) and therefore not easy to give up or modify. But anyone is better off learning to do this, and if going cold turkey is not possible, drastically limiting and cutting back should be everyone's health goal. In short, we have to change the way we look at food and not simply a reward for good behavior. And finally, don't be fooled by the skinny person who can seem to eat anything and not gain weight—as their innards suffer damage just as much.

An Addendum on Vitamins

This addendum is part of the nutrition chapter for the reason that there exists much controversy in the medical community concerning them. I hope to shed some light as to why the controversy exists in the first place. To begin, the body operates nutritionally on a chemical basis, and on that basis, certain substances have been isolated and given the name vitamins, as being vital to life. These substances are found in the food we eat, and it can be shown that various vitamins affect the operation and health of the body. A typical example is iodine, which is found in abundance in seafood. However, what happens when the body doesn't get enough as not everyone likes seafood. Well, one thing you are likely develop is goiter, a spare tire-like swelling around the neck. Many years ago, the government required iodine to be added to salt and thus the name iodized salt, which you are probably familiar with.

We can go down the vitamin list and note all the bodily functions associated with them. We've all heard of patients given vitamin B12 shots for weakness due to an illness. So we can pose the question, if vitamins are necessary for life and health, where's the controversy? And, we might add, try not getting any which would mean eating nothing but tofu for a week, and see how good you would feel. (But as they say, don't try this at home.)

To answer the question on controversy, it is that popping vitamins without knowing their effect, as some can be harmful if too much is ingested, can be an expensive and dangerous proposition. And since we are all different from each other in DNA mix, we all don't need the same amounts. Also, it is felt that vitamins without the food vehicle to carry them are as not effective. Some believe not effective at all.

So this leaves us with a conundrum: do we vitaminize or not? Once again, the answer (and you saw this coming) is eat a balanced diet, and do a little study of your own on what foods supply what vitamins. It's not that hard. Much information is right on the Internet. Secondly, ask your physician, using blood testing, plus observation, to assess your vitamin needs. And particularly ask for a vitamin D level test as this vitamin is closely linked to your immune system.

Other than a specifically prescribe vitamin, the middle ground of safety and balance is take a multiple vitamins with food once a day. In these times, this is generally what's recommended.

And one last point, try to get good-quality vitamins as some might be manufactured under questionable sources, which is another reason why vitamin supplements are frowned on. Also don't adopt the nefarious rule "if a little is good, a lot has to be better." Look at the RDA on the label (recommended daily allowance) and work within those parameters. Keep in mind that a person's size and weight have a lot to do with what's needed, and you are really supposed to be supplementing what you should be getting from the food you eat. Once again, common sense goes a long way.

Alcohol, Tobacco, and Caregiving

In a not so indirect way, alcohol and tobacco are a part of caregiving. I don't think you'll find too many people today, with all that is known about the harmful effects of smoking, dispute the fact that it is harmful and deadly—perhaps as many has those flat earthers who think it still is. Less and less people do it, and many of those would like to quit (a good idea if you are one of them). But there are caregivers who are caring for a smoker. If not a family member, you can politely ask them not to smoke when you're there (you may get fired, but you'd be better off not inhaling even secondhand smoke (the old myth that it is not harmful). However, if you your patient is a spouse or family member, your job may not be so easy.

Smokers rationalize in a number of ways, and I think I've heard them all. And probably so have you. These are as follows: "I know so and so who smoked and lived to be ninety-five" or "Nobody's ever proven smoking will kill you" or "I've done it too long to quit" or "I know it's bad and I'd like to quit—maybe next week" or "I hope you never start."

My recommendation is to try, in as kind a way as you can, to let your patient know that you care about them and that you want to keep them around and you know smoking is bad for their recovery, healing, and general health (not to mention your own). If you do this sympathetically, you may get through; some caregivers actually do.

As to alcohol, many of the same things can be said, but unlike smoking, alcohol is still socially acceptable. Usually, the rule of thumb is one drink a day (of several ounces). And of course, it depends on what you're drinking. Hard liquor is far more potent and harmful than a glass of wine (and red wine is known to have some health benefits). However, alcohol is still a chemical that the body is better off not ingesting. A beverage very low in alcohol would be the most desirable way to have a drink, such as low-alcohol fruit drinks. But for someone who prefers scotch, rum, a martini, the former would not satisfy. So moderation is called for.

Having said these things as a kind of lefthanded defense for having a drink, it is part of the social fabric. But at the same time, it impairs judgment and driving and a lot sooner than many realize. I personally believe one is better off not smoking or drinking, but it is a personal choice. However, as a caregiver, you may encounter the "secret" or a heavy drinker that is sneaking drinks and hiding their liquor. My own dad, sadly, did this. It destroyed his liver, and he passed at age fifty-two. His autopsy revealed every other organ was as a man in his twenties! What made him drink? To this day, I don't know, but I do know his family lost him way too soon—and alcohol was the poison.

Many caregivers may be caring for someone despondent and alcohol may be their comfort and escape. So for obvious reasons, you must be on the lookout for this.

Everyone has a free will so if an individual insists on drinking to excess or smoking; you cannot throw them in jail. What you can do is try to help them to see and modify behavior for as low health impact as possible.

Incontinence—Accidents
and Cleanup

As a caregiver, one of the more unpleasant things you might find yourself having to deal with is incontinence and the resultant clean-ups of patient and environment sometimes necessary.

In normal function, this is another area not usually given much thought until one has to. Conditions resulting from aging or the debilitation resulting from an illness itself, as in Parkinson's, produces a life management situation that must be handled.

The first thing to be aware of is the embarrassment the patient suffers. It is an affront at times to one's dignity. One comes to feel they must never be a few steps from a bathroom. And sometimes even at that, a sudden urgency or unawareness can result in an uncontrolled voiding. And of course, such an occurrence must be dealt with.

Fortunately, there are garments and products designed to be worn to help with this problem, and they do a good job, although not always 100 percent. So as a professional caregiver or a spouse, this is another one of the more unpleasant aspects of the job.

It should be pointed out that this is not a terminal condition—unless it is a hospice situation. So one must be prepared to deal with this for perhaps a considerable stretch of time in one's life.

Referring back to Parkinson's, because so many bodily functions are affected by it, it is not unusual for a patient to experience incontinence to some degree. There are medications that can help, but to what degree depends on the patient. This condition should be brought to the attention of the appropriate physician (usually a urologist), and from that point, recommendations can be made.

Urinary incontinence can also signal an infection and not necessarily connected to the main illness. But left untreated, they can be very serious. Also bowel incontinence can signal something just as serious and should be evaluated and not dismissed.

If you're thinking, "I can deal with anything but not adult incontinence," ask yourself, if you've raised a child from babyhood, you've dealt with that. And while not pleasant in the least, love can find a way to handle that too.

The "Placement" Separation

Sometimes, caregiving a spouse ends not because the loved one has passed but because the level of care required can no longer be provided by the spouse. Often at this age level or required caregiving, one or the other partner cannot handle or provide care without detriment to one or the other. When this point is reached, the next step is assisted living for the party in need. However, it really should be looked at as assisted living for both parties as when the one in most need receives help, it is helping to lift the burden off the other.

When assisted living is needed, it can be provided in several ways: (1) in home limited daytime hours, (2) in home 24-7, or (3) assisted living facility. We'll briefly discuss all three.

1. In home limited. This simply means a caregiver assistant helps with the chores and the needs of the patient a limited and designated number of hours. This can vary and be adjusted to the needs of the situation. Often a good, less expensive solution to receiving the extra care needed. Many companies specialize in this such as Visiting Angels that can handle everything from cooking, shopping, cleaning, getting patient to doctors, etc. You may be surprised at what they can handle and are equipped and trained to do.

2. In home 24-7. This is a next step and a more expensive one. Plus it changes the privacy dynamic of the home. Not everyone is comfortable with this type of arrangement, plus your living quarters need to provide a bedroom, preferably separated from the general living quarters and better yet with a separate entrance. While few homes are set up this way, it does make having a stranger in the home constantly

a bit easier. But at the very least, a bedroom and nearby separate or extra bathroom is needed for this to work in as least awkward way as possible.

3. Assisted living facility. Sometimes this is the only alternative. Different types and levels of these exist from a couple to share or just the spouse alone. They are more expensive per month and are most economical if the couple can move in together. This is not always preferable or possible for a host of reasons. If it is just for the one spouse, consider a facility that rents via typical lease, so you don't have to liquidate all to access this type of facility. Obviously, while time permits, investigate and visit what's available where you live. But in any case, choose one where you can visit regularly as this is a separation of sorts and not an easy move or decision.

And be prepared for a large emotional whack as if your marriage is close; it will be. Even if you visit daily, you must still return to an empty house, and I assure you it will not be easy. At this time of things, you will need God's comfort and assurance it's only temporary and the best is yet to come—as the scriptures assure us.

The Exhaustion Factor

The fact that caregiving is exhausting is well established and has been referred to a number of times in this book. But if you are new to caregiving professionally speaking or have recently become one due to family or marital life developments, you are just beginning to learn just how exhausting and draining it is.

There are reasons for this being so, and before you start asking yourself, "What's wrong with me? Why am I so drained and tired?" we'll consider the factors in the exhaustion syndrome. To start with, there are three levels of exhaustion: physical, mental/emotional, and spiritual. And when all three hit together, well, that can and does set someone back on their heels, so to speak. And if you become exhausted to the point of despair and hopelessness, you are in a state that is serious, and while in this state, you cannot administer your caregiving assignment properly.

One very big underlying reason this state develops is due to the relentlessness of caregiving. If you are caregiving for a spouse or a child or a parent, especially a spouse or a child, you are in a 24-7 situation. Caregiving demands so much of one's time, energy, and response, especially when dealing with dementia in all forms, that you as the caregiver literally become burned out. And when one is in this position, it is like being a trapped animal with no escape or, to use a better analogy, one imprisoned. And as this state progresses, one can literally lose their identity and purposeful living.

Which brings up the question whether one can literally live wholly for the welfare of another? And this point is raised to spotlight whether even for a child or mate. Well, many have subjugated themselves to just such a task. And again raises the point of the difficulties that arise in caregiving.

One comment you hear frequently is "I have little or no time to myself, and I'm too worn out to make much use of it anyway." Another is "I've lost contact with all my friends" or "I have no life other than caregiving." Yes, caregiving causes one to sacrifice much. Even professionally because while you get to leave your assignment (unless you're a live-in one), you still return to your home duties, and this may include caring for a family of your own.

So the bottom line is you are going to get tired. And to counteract this, you will need to find activities both physical, mental, and spiritual to counteract this. The key word is counteract and renew. I'll list them, but it will be up to you to apply and balance what fits.

1. Hobbies of your choice and interest (in my case, playing my musical instruments), and these can be as varied as there are interests and time.
2. Proper sleep and rest.
3. Proper nutrition.
4. Exercise. Here some home equipment can help. Examples are as follows: stairclimbing, forty-five-degree pushups in a counter or chair, squats, walking if you can get outdoors.
5. Calling or e-mailing friends and relatives.
6. Keeping a diary.
7. Cooking to the extent and ability.
8. Occasional home help. If you can afford it, there are organizations that can provide this and thus give you a break to shop, meet with friends, or a round of golf.
9. Prayer. Pray for God's sustaining help and acceptance in your role and don't neglect this area.

Yes, caregiving is a most difficult role, and two things you don't want to become is bitter and loss of personhood. It doesn't have to happen, but you must be alert and acknowledge that it can and thus take steps to ensure it doesn't.

Handling Guilt

Guilt—an energy- and life-robbing emotion that often accompanies caregiving. It is a terrible nagging mental and emotional state that persists in someone who has lost a loved one that they were caring for. This is most often true and strongest in losing a parent, child, or perhaps most acutely, a spouse. It is bad enough to be grieving for a lost loved one, but to be bearing guilt on top of that is—and there is no other way to put it—just an awful mental and emotional state to suffer in.

What are the causes of this guilt? Is it legitimate and normal to have it? And is there anything that can be done about it?

To start with, guilt is a feeling that arises from believing or thinking you have wronged someone or that you are responsible for what has happened. Well, if out of neglect or maliciousness you have, then you should feel guilt. However, the guilt one feels in caregiving is thinking one could have, should have, or would have done more. In short, it is blaming yourself for your loved one's passing or, at best, being placed in a nursing facility.

It can be debated whether the guilt and mourning we are experiencing is out of sadness, altruism, or selfishness for the passing or the placing, but perhaps, as so many human emotions, it is a mixture and a combination of many. The debate can center around whether one is selfish for mourning one's loss (and why wouldn't we mourn over that?) or whether being deprived of the loving presence of another just plain leaves a large hole in one's psyche. But if one has loved to the best of one's abilities being imperfect in an imperfect world—even with God's acknowledged blessing and help—then one has to come to rest in the state and belief that it is love that wins this debate.

However, often one will go over and over in their mind things like "How could I have missed that?" or "I should have seen that and told the doctor" or still "I should have caught them when they stumbled too close to the stairs." Thoughts like this can become a nightmare on a loop playing over and over and can rob others around you of the best of your presence, ruin your sleep, and possibly your very health.

What is the answer to this state, and is there any help for it? There is, but first you will have to ask yourself several questions—and perhaps more than once. And if the answers are hopefully what they should be, you will come to a state of peace concerning your loss.

Before we tackle these questions though, you must understand and accept a period of grieving. This is normal, expected, and biblical. It is the unending state of guilt we want to deal with.

The first question is "Did you truly love that person, and do you intensely miss them?"

The second question is "If they were still here or with you, would you still wish to be their caregiver despite the known hardships?"

The third question is "To the best of your understanding and ability, did you do the best you could?"

The fourth question is "Do you acknowledge the fact that you are not omnipotent and are a limited human being?"

The fifth question is "Do you believe in and acknowledge the sovereignty, timing, and will of God?"

The sixth question is "Do you believe God loved whom you loved?"

The seventh question is "Do you believe God loves and cares for you?"

The eight question is "Do you believe God has promised an exceedingly complete and full restoration of all things and of those who know and love Him?"

If you've been able to answer yes to all the questions, you are in a good place to be receiving spiritual comfort to have your guilt removed and to go on loving and helping others and those around you. Remembering the God who loved and created you loses nothing. Jesus is, after all, the Good Shepherd.

Conclusion and Patient Release

It's always great then when the patient receives the OK and all clear to resume normal life. Many special relationships have been forged due to caregiving, even marriages. And often, the relationship that ensued is missed when the care is no longer needed.

If there is a lesson to be learned from the caregiving need and function, it is that we are all related through God who made us. We are, in fact, all brothers and sisters who will care for and love one another and share our love and interests. The scripture "Look not only on your own things but on the things of others" (Philippians 2:4) stated this principle clearly. In short, we are to be instruments of helping one another to fulfill ours and others dreams and to become what God intends for each of us to be. If this is the lesson, it is a great one indeed. The second great commandment of "love thy neighbor as thyself" says it as directly and forcefully as it can be said.

When growing up and in my college years during one of my many conversations with my dad, he commented, "The attitude I think is most awful says, 'The hell with you, I'm all right'" (his exact words). At the time, I didn't understand it in depth the way I do today, but as with all his comments and admonitions, it has stayed with me.

Not a churchgoer but I marvel at his spiritual wisdom about so many things. However, I also want to hasten to add that I do not advocate nonchurchgoing or shunning of organized religion(s), but rather I am pointing out that spiritual wisdom comes in many ways.

Today, I understand his comment to mean when you express the attitude he condemned, you are really saying, "Me first" and "I don't really care if you are not doing well." This is a condemnable attitude and certainly not a godly one. When we come to understand

113

tne sovereignty of God as the singular Creator of everything and that He loves His Creation and commands that we love it too, why we can do nothing less. When you get down to it, it is completely logical. And it explains the scripture, "He who hates his brother is [in reality] a murderer" (1 John 3:15) as in that person's heart, he/she would be quite happy if that individual never even existed. A harsh statement, yes, but consider the meaning. Get out of the gray area because with God, you don't get gray but direct unvarnished truth. And as an aside, the gray area of thought and attitude is where liberalism resides—and realize that God always takes things to the heart of the matter. In short, if you love something, you will care for it, and if you don't, you will discard it at some point.

Sometimes our emotions make us want to do just that—to run the other way—but our godly free will says, "No! I won't run. I will help." Now you've put your finger on where the spirit of caregiving resides.

So What Have We Learned?

At first, you might think this is a strange chapter to include in a book of this kind. But it isn't really.

God regards us in our journey through life and asks the question, "All right, up to this point, what have you learned?" Humans often ask the question about life this way: "How much have I achieved or gotten in wealth, prestige, or power?" Right away, we see that God must look at life differently than we do—and He does. The old adage "you can't take it with you" holds for all this so called wealth, prestige, power, and possessions.

Why does God ask the question this way? If we don't take our earthly possessions when we depart, is there anything we do take? The answer to that question is yes, we take the spiritual truths we have accepted and embraced. This is what is meant by the scriptural admonition to "lay up treasure in Heaven where moth, dust and rust, do not corrupt" (Matthew 6:19). In short, that which is spiritual, immortal, and indestructible.

In this regard, life events and circumstances are great teachers. It has been observed, circumstances don't just cause—they reveal. They ultimately teach us what's most important. The Bible is clear about that, in that we are to love God with all we've got and our neighbor as ourselves.

It comes down to this: we all need love, kindness, and caring from God and from each other. There are individuals who might dispute this thinking in that they conduct their lives as self-sufficient islands. But they are very mistaken, and one must hope they, at some point, come to see this.

The thing then in life that can teach and reinforce this principle is caregiving. And the treasure we take with us is the realization and the praising of the fact that we are all related to God who made us. There is great comfort in this. It is, as the old hymn states, "the tie that binds."

My career choice, after considering New Jersey State Police, music, and astrophysics, was musician/teacher. Though I've never lost my interest and regard for the other two, I believe I made the right choice. But I've also learned something else. Learning never stops, nor should it. And one should not limit one's acquiring as much as possible, knowledge about any and all things. And it is hoped the reader will see it that way as well.

Along these lines, in my early twenties, my trombone teacher in Philadelphia, Dr. Donald S. Reinhardt, remarked in one of my lessons, in his words, "I never gave a lesson that I didn't get one." I've always hung on to that because it turns out to be so true. Everything about life is a teacher including teaching itself.

Have you noticed that people who win enormous sums of money in lotteries often wind up with many headaches and not in a good place? I'm sure when they learned they had won this fortune, they rejoiced. After all, isn't money supposed to bring all desired things into one's life? Well, if you mean greedy, entitled, expectant relatives, friends, salespeople, and just plain not knowing how to manage such a large sum, and perhaps blowing most, if not all, of it, then the answer would be yes.

After one has bought everything in sight, what's left? Who's going to sail and maintain that yacht—another expense. And that accountant's fee for managing your wealth. But before going further, I'm not putting down wealth but rather pointing out that wealth alone does not bring nor guarantee happiness, wisdom, or common sense.

There's the story of the suddenly wealthy couple who decided to take a world cruise. When they returned, a friend asked, "How was it?" They remarked, "Oh, it was great, and next week we're going someplace else!" That ultimate question "What does it profit a man to gain the whole world but lose one's soul, and what will he give in exchange for it?" (Matthew 16:26).

You see the point. The joy, true joy in life, is God and others. I began to see this truth some time ago as a musician when it occurred to me that a musician needs someone to play for—in short, an audience. It's giving to others really, and we all have something to give and receive. A musician has that to give, an artist a visual creation and expression, a chef a wonderful meal, and God, incredible vistas and life itself, as well as Himself.

But back to caregiving. What is given and what is received? The answer, I'm sure, is as varied as the circumstances involved. And at first, and perhaps for years, you might not know or find out, particularly as a professional serving clients on a much more temporary basis. Within a family or a mate, however, the answer is or will be more immediate and obvious. But as things move along (life), you will get inklings and realizations.

As a music teacher in public school, now retired, I will occasionally meet or run into a former student—sometimes from thirty or more years ago. It is always nice to hear that they loved what they were taught and felt you were a good teacher. I've even had the pleasure of working professionally with a student of mine, who, years ago I taught as a beginner and who are now themselves a professional musician. That, as the saying goes, is reward enough. However, behind that remark and compliment is something deeper. And that something they are expressing is that they felt love and regard extended to them. That, frankly, matters a whole lot more. God says in scripture that whatever you do for someone, you are doing also to God Himself! A deep and remarkable fundamental as, in reverse, as you do these things, it is God helping you to do them.

Behind caregiving is that very principle. God is overjoyed when we learn and embrace that. "Look not only on your own things, but on the things of others" (Philippians 2:4). Things here means all of life's cares, concerns, projects, and interests. Some lessons are learned the hard way over a period of time. However, caregiving is often a crash course—especially with a child, family, or mate.

Finally, from time to time, one looks back on where one has been in one's life and takes stock, which we are inevitably as humans prompted to do. It is at these times one often says, this (whatever "this" might be) has changed me. I'm now a different person. We often put it this way: I've grown.

Hollywood, on occasion, gets it right. The much-revered movie *It's a Wonderful Life*, starring Jimmy Stewart, is such an example. Through miraculous happenings, a man is transported to a life he thought he was seeking, which as it turns out, was wrong, and he realizes it. When he comes to his senses, he cries out to God (through an angel), and he is transported back to his former life and his family. I believe this happens to all of us in many ways and God is very clever and loving in how He accomplishes this. Perhaps not as dramatically as in that movie but God meeting us spiritually where we need to be met.

At this point, I encourage you to look back on your own life and think of the individuals who helped you along the way to become who and what you are today. I personally can think of ten that were pivotal for me in a large way, and many more friends who shared my interests and goals. I can think of one individual—my first guitar teacher, a George Brandon, a brilliant humble man, who my dad would remind me from time to time that I should thank God for him every night "because he saved you" (musically speaking), and my dad was so right.

Today, how many can you sight that perhaps you were key to their progress and success in life? You may not know the answer to the second part—at least not yet—but when all is made known I'm sure you'll see you've been fitted yourself and have assisted others to be fitted into the mosaic of God's eternal plan.

About the Author

The book you are about to read came about through Mr. Tegeder's experience caring for his wife who suffers from Parkinson's. It is written from the heart and from a godly perspective. At the time this book was written Mr. and Mrs. Tegeder have been married for fifty-one years, and Mr. Tegeder has seen his wife progress from a very mild form of this disease to a point where the effects have eroded his wife's capabilities in so many areas of daily living.

Though Mr. Tegeder's professional training and degrees are in the area of music, his degree also included training in physics, psychology, chemistry, and premed biology and physiology providing the background to assimilate and present the caregiving role from many aspects.

It is hoped that the reader will be helped to understand and cope with a very difficult life assignment, using what is available and known medically, with the spiritual side with love foremost and at the center.

And it is his belief that one will come through this difficult life experience a better, deeper, more caring, and understanding person and, in the end, be moved closer to God.